Helen Senderovich
Megan Vierhout

Integrated End of Life Care in Dementia

Helen Senderovich
Megan Vierhout

Integrated End of Life Care in Dementia

Recognizing Dementia as a Life-Limiting Illness and The Benefits of Implementing Palliative Care

Scholars' Press

Imprint

Any brand names and product names mentioned in this book are subject to trademark, brand or patent protection and are trademarks or registered trademarks of their respective holders. The use of brand names, product names, common names, trade names, product descriptions etc. even without a particular marking in this work is in no way to be construed to mean that such names may be regarded as unrestricted in respect of trademark and brand protection legislation and could thus be used by anyone.

Cover image: www.ingimage.com

Publisher:
Scholars' Press
is a trademark of
Dodo Books Indian Ocean Ltd. and OmniScriptum S.R.L publishing group

120 High Road, East Finchley, London, N2 9ED, United Kingdom
Str. Armeneasca 28/1, office 1, Chisinau MD-2012, Republic of Moldova, Europe

ISBN: 978-620-5-52185-4

Copyright © Helen Senderovich, Megan Vierhout
Copyright © 2023 Dodo Books Indian Ocean Ltd. and OmniScriptum S.R.L publishing group

Table of Contents

LIST OF ABBREVIATIONS 1
INTRODUCTION 2
CASE STUDY 3
WHAT IS DEMENTIA? 6
WHAT IS PALLIATIVE CARE? 8
INTEGRATION OF PALLIATIVE CARE IN DEMENTIA 9
SYMPTOM MANAGEMENT 12
PALLIATIVE CONTINUOUS DEEP SEDATION AND MEDICAL ASSISTANCE IN DYING 21
DEPRESCRIBING IN DEMENTIA 23
MODELS OF PALLIATIVE CARE 33
ILLNESS TRAJECTORY AND PROGRESS 36
BENEFITS OF PALLIATIVE CARE 39
RECOMMENDATIONS FOR PALLIATIVE CARE 43
RESOURCE AVAILABILITY 45
AGE-RELATED INEQUALITIES AND ACCESSIBILITY 46
HEALTH SYSTEM IMPLICATIONS 47
KNOWLEDGE TRANSLATION 48
FUTURE RESEARCH 50
CONCLUSION 52
REFERENCES 54

List of Abbreviations

Abbreviation	Definition
ACP	advance care planning
CDS	continuous deep sedation
CPR	cardiopulmonary resuscitation
EMBED-Care	Empowering Better End-of-Life Dementia Care
GDS	Global Deterioration Scale for Assessment of Primary Degenerative Dementia
GP	general practitioner
IMPACT	Implementation of quality indicators in Palliative Care sTudy)
KPS	Karnofsky Performance Scale
KT	knowledge translation
LTC	long term care
MAiD	medical assistance in dying
MMSE	Mini-Mental State Examination
MoCA	Montreal Cognitive Assessment
NMDA	N-methyl-D-aspartate
PACS-LAC	Pain Assessment Checklist for Seniors with Limited Ability to Communicate
PAINAD	Pain Assessment in Advanced Dementia
PC	palliative care
PIG	Proactive Identification Guidance
PPS	Palliative Performance Scale
RASS	Richmond Agitation-Sedation Scale
SQ	surprise question

Introduction

Dementia is a progressive neurological condition primarily involving cognitive impairment and a decline in the level of functioning of affected patients. Over 55 million individuals worldwide live with dementia, and due to the increasing proportion of older people, it is expected that this number will rise to 78 million by 2030, and 139 million by 2050 (World Health Organization, 2022). The rapid increase in the aging population highlights the importance of management of this debilitating disease. Despite this prevalence, dementia is not a part of aging, and can be complex and challenging to treat as the course of progression is unique to each patient. Reliable tools for prognostication in dementia are lacking, however patients with advanced disease may experience death from a sudden event, such as a fracture (Murray et al., 2005). Not recognizing dementia as a terminal illness complicates the establishment of effective care models, and leaves patients and caregivers with a limited understanding of disease trajectory. As the symptoms of dementia are multifaceted, some including pain, dyspnea, frailty, cognitive impairment, anxiety, and effects on emotional management and social behaviour, patient distress and caregiver burden are paramount concerns. There is a need for personalized care to optimize quality of life for patients suffering with dementia, as well as their caregivers. Palliative care (PC) is a multidisciplinary approach that requires the expertise of various healthcare professionals, depending on the needs of the patient. In dementia, this may include neurological, psychosocial and physical support. As this type of care emphasizes a patient-centred approach that is uniquely tailored to the individual, it has multiple perceived benefits for integration in complex conditions such as dementia.

Case Study

Mrs. A is an 80-year-old woman who was living at home with her husband, daughter, and son-in law. Mrs. A's daughter began to notice increased forgetfulness and frustration in Mrs. A. She had difficulty with everyday activities such as meal preparation, and was unable to concentrate on tasks that were a part of her routine for many years. Her family also noted behaviours out of Mrs. A's usual personality, including sudden bursts of anger or sadness. Mrs. A's family became increasingly concerned and made an appointment to see her family doctor, Dr. X. Following his assessment, Dr. X informed Mrs. A and her family that she was likely experiencing early symptoms of dementia, and referred her to a geriatric outpatient clinic at the local hospital. Mrs. A's past medical history included osteoarthritis, chronic back pain, hypertension, and coronary artery disease. Her medications included statins, calcium channel blockers, acetaminophen, and multivitamins.

Dr. Y, who was the geriatrician at the clinic, conducted a full evaluation of Mrs. A and confirmed the diagnosis of dementia. Dr. Y explained to Mrs. A and her family that although there is no cure for dementia, there were multiple management options. He discussed the role of PC in dementia management and informed them about the availability of the PC program offered at the hospital, which included home visits. Naturally, Mrs. A and her family expressed fear and hesitation, but agreed to have a PC consultation. The team explored the benefits of PC in dementia, and how early integration of PC can impact her quality of life. Mrs. A and her family decided to move forward with introducing home PC with monthly home visits by Dr. Z.

During the home visits, Dr. Z educated Mrs. X and her family on the trajectory of dementia, and helped to create a comprehensive advance care plan that was individually tailored to Mrs. A's values, beliefs, and preferences. Mrs. A was able to make important decisions regarding her care.

She communicated her worries surrounding overwhelming her family with her care, and expressed her desire to be institutionalized in a facility when her disease advanced. Dr. Z prescribed Mrs. A an analgesic for managing her chronic muscle pain, and arranged regular visits by a personal support worker from the community to assist Mrs. A with cooking and cleaning.

As time elapsed, Mrs. A's symptoms progressed from mild to moderate in the next two years. Her cognitive awareness markedly declined. She was forgetting the names of her family members, and care at home became challenging as she was often agitated. Mrs. A's family, together with Dr. Z, decided that it was in Mrs. A's best interest to admit her to the long-term care facility associated with the local hospital, so her care needs could be met. In the long-term care facility, Mrs. A began to receive more intensive PC. A speech language pathologist and dietician worked together to create a feeding plan to minimize choking hazard due to progressive swallowing difficulties associated with dysphagia, and ensure adequate nutrition. Mrs. A was prescribed risperidone with received verbal consent from her proxy to control agitation. Additionally, she was prescribed an anti-emetic to manage her nausea, and her acetaminophen prescription was maximized to adequately manage increased pain. Her family visited her regularly and she participated in therapeutic recreation activities, including music therapy and bingo.

Over the next year, Mrs. A's health continued to deteriorate. The health care team, in consultation with the family, decided to discontinue many of Mrs. A's long-term medications, such as statins, antihypertensives, and multivitamins, as the impression was that she would not benefit from them anymore. She was no longer able to communicate and was observed to be agitated. As time progressed, she was noted to be declining further, and started to approach end of life. Her Palliative Performance Scale and Karnofsky Performance Scale scores were evaluated and found to be at 10%. As she was noted to be approaching end of life, she was transferred to the

PC ward in the hospital where one week later she died peacefully surrounded by her family and loved ones.

What is Dementia?

Dementia is a chronic and progressive neurological condition that affects the brain. The hallmark of this syndrome is cognitive impairment, classified by a decrease in the previous level of functioning of the individual. Dementia results in impairment of functional abilities and may or may not be accompanied by behavioural and psychological disruptions in some patients. Higher cortical functions, such as memory, comprehension, and orientation, are affected. Deterioration in emotional control, motivation, and social behaviour may also be observed (National Institute for Health and Care Excellence, 2018). These signs and symptoms were observed in the presented case study of Mrs. A, where she experienced progressive forgetfulness and memory loss, with eventual onset of agitation and loss of awareness.

Over 55 million people worldwide are currently living with dementia, with approximately 10 million new cases diagnosed each year (World Health Organization, 2022). Despite a wide array of affected individuals, dementia is not a part of aging, and the course of progression of the disease is unique to each patient. There is a myriad of types of dementia, such as Alzheimer's dementia, dementia of Parkinson's disease, vascular dementia, frontotemporal dementia, Lewy body dementia, and mixed dementia. Among these types, Alzheimer's dementia is the most prevalent, accounting for approximately 60-70% of all dementia cases worldwide (National Institute for Health and Care Excellence, 2018; World Health Organization, 2022). This type of dementia specifically is classified by the aggregation of beta amyloid plaques (NIH National Institute on Aging, 2017). Overall, due to its complexity and lack of effective treatment options, the management of dementia presents multifaceted challenges for healthcare providers.

Dementia not only significantly affects the individual, but also alters the lives of the family and caregivers of those affected with this disease. Quality of life is an established outcome measure for patients with dementia

(Hoe et al., 2009). It is crucial to determine management options and care plans that consider achieving the best quality of life for patients and caregivers faced with the disease.

What is Palliative Care?

The World Health Organization defines PC as "an approach that improves the quality of life of patients (adults and children) and their families who are facing problems associated with life-threatening illness" (World Health Organization, 2020). This type of care aims to provide patients with the services they require to achieve comfort and adequate management of their symptoms. PC encompasses a patient-centred approach and focuses on treating the patient as a whole, rather than solely focusing on the disease. Dementia is often not viewed as a life-threatening illness, which complicates the timely integration of PC for those affected with this disease (Hughes et al., 2007). The current standard of care does not include the integration of a PC team when a patient is diagnosed with dementia (Murphy et al., 2016). However, PC can be beneficial in the management of dementia as it can improve the quality of life of the patient and family. PC also employs a multidisciplinary healthcare team to meet the multiple needs of patients with dementia, including physical, psychological, and social support of those affected and their caregivers.

Integration of Palliative Care in Dementia

Advance Care Planning and End of Life Conversations

Advance care planning (ACP) involves creating an individualized care plan and mapping out potential future decisions for a patient's care. The patient should be educated on disease development and trajectory, what to expect down the road, prognosis, the available treatment options and their success rates, and the array of decisions that may need to be made. From there, a care plan can be constructed that incorporates the patient's values, beliefs, and preferences, which provides the healthcare team with direction, and allows patients to have control over disease management. Some of the possible decisions that ACP includes are cardiopulmonary resuscitation (CPR), ventilator use, artificial nutrition, artificial hydration, and comfort care (NIH National Institute on Aging, 2022). ACP is different from general care planning and employs disease progression (Harrison Dening et al., 2019). The benefits of ACP are especially evident in the context of dementia, where the patient often loses cognition and may be deemed incapable of informed decision making. At the same time, ACP is complex in the setting of dementia as there is limited evidence on how to engage dementia patients and their families in this process (van der Steen, 2021).

Some patients with dementia are still able to participate in the decision-making process, and those who are still able to understand can be consulted to create care plans outlining their wishes and preferences. Fortunately, Mrs. A was able to participate in decision-making regarding her care while creating a plan with Dr. Z and her family. When the illness has progressed, families are often put in the position to make decisions for the patient regarding end of life care, and the patient's proxy should be appointed. Timing of these discussions can pose challenges. Should the patient be informed about the illness trajectory and educated about what to expect so an informed decision can be made while they still have decision-making capacity? Or would this be too overwhelming and only complicate matters? Berrio and Levesque (1996) have outlined various barriers for ACP from the patient's perspective, which include: a knowledge gap on ACP, difficulty of discussing and accepting 'bad' news, procrastination, depending on family to make decisions, belief that a lawyer is needed for completion of paperwork, fatalism, fear of 'signing life away', and fear of not receiving treatment (Berrio & Levesque, 1996). Harrison Dening added dementia-specific barriers to this list, including: the lack of acknowledgement of dementia as a terminal disease, patients' loss of decision-making capacity in earlier stages of the disease, caregivers' unawareness on disease trajectory in dementia, lack of confidence in healthcare professionals and challenges associated with initiating goals of care discussions in dementia patients, and failure to appoint someone to manage ongoing ACP (Harrison Dening, 2018; Harrison Dening et al., 2019). It may also be difficult for patients to fully grasp symptoms associated with more advanced disease. A qualitative study exploring the perspectives of patients with mild dementia on oral intake in later stages of dementia revealed that many people struggled to relate these issues with dementia progression (Anantapong et al., 2021).

One of the aims of PC is to initiate early conversations addressing the patient's goals for end of life care. Thorough communication between patients, family members, and healthcare providers is crucial in this setting. It has been reported that knowledge surrounding PC is an important factor in the willingness of patients and families to accept PC (Cardenas et al., 2022; Myint et al., 2021), which emphasizes the need for early and clear communication in the setting of life-limiting illness. As reported by Sampson et al. (2011), there may also be reluctance from patients and family members to face ACP discussion (Sampson et al., 2011). This may be related to some of the barriers mentioned above, such as difficulty discussing approaching end of life care, lack of education of the public, and healthcare providers who may not feel comfortable initiating this conversation, which is frequently linked to lack of knowledge about the disease trajectory of dementia. This could possibly be minimized by timely discussion during earlier stages of the illness regarding diagnosis and what to expect with patients and caregivers. Additionally, healthcare provider education on ACP is a crucial factor in its successful implementation. Hendriks et al. (2017) reported that despite a "do not hospitalize order", 21% of long-term care (LTC) facility patients with dementia were indeed hospitalized (Hendriks et al., 2017). This stresses the importance of healthcare provider education in the timely revisitation of patients' ACP and goals of care.

Symptom Management

Dementia is a disease of inevitably progressive nature, however, the progression and course of onset of symptoms is unique to each individual. Since there are no curative or effective treatment options for this disease, it is imperative to focus on symptom management in order to maximize quality of life for patients with dementia. Additionally, one of the main pillars of PC is prioritizing symptom relief. As the disease progresses, patients may require additional support and different forms of care. Symptom management intensifies at the end of life (Hendriks et al., 2015). It is often difficult to assess the PC needs of dementia patients, especially in a standardised manner, and thus looking to symptoms documented in the routine care of patients can be useful (Schunk et al., 2021). It is key to employ effective symptom management throughout illness trajectory of dementia and introduce PC as part of practice in early stages.

Pain

50% of all dementia patients worldwide and 72% of patients over the age of 85 experience regular pain (Achterberg et al., 2013). Despite this prevalence, pain remains a challenging and poorly understood symptom in those suffering with dementia. The effect of changes in neuropathology and decreased communication capacity are issues that may complicate pain management in dementia patients (Achterberg et al., 2013). This not only raises challenges in the treatment of pain, but also creates barriers for adequate assessment. As a result, pain is undertreated in patients with dementia (Sarbacker, 2014).

Pain in dementia is primarily musculoskeletal (Sarbacker, 2014), as it was seen with Mrs. A who was suffering from chronic back pain and was prescribed acetaminophen. Pain may manifest in this population via behavioural issues, including agitation and wandering (Sarbacker, 2014). Although the current standard of care for pain assessment in dementia is patient self-report (such as visual analog scales and Numeric Rating Scale), this is often only practical in mild and moderate dementia (Sarbacker, 2014). In advanced dementia, observation scales are more suitable as this population has lost the ability to communicate. Examples of observational tools include the Pain Assessment Checklist for Seniors with Limited Ability to Communicate (PACS-LAC), the Observational Pain Behavior Tool, and the Pain Assessment in Advanced Dementia (PAINAD) scale (Figure 1) (Sarbacker, 2014; Warden et al., 2003). The selection of proper medications for pain control can be challenging. Typical therapies include analgesics (opioid, non-opioid, adjuvant), corticosteroids, and calcitonin (Sarbacker, 2014).

Pain Assessment in Advanced Dementia (PAINAD)

	0	1	2	Score
Breathing Independent of vocalization	Normal	Occasional labored breathing. Short period of hyperventilation	Noisy labored breathing. Long period of hyperventilation. Cheyne-Stokes respirations.	
Negative vocalization	None	Occasional moan or groan. Low-level speech with a negative or disapproving quality.	Repeated troubled calling out. Loud moaning or groaning. Crying.	
Facial expression	Smiling, or inexpressive	Sad. Frightened. Frown	Facial grimacing	
Body language	Relaxed	Tense. Distressed pacing. Fidgeting.	Rigid. Fists clenched. Knees pulled up. Pulling or pushing away. Striking out.	
Consolability	No need to console	Distracted or reassured by voice or touch.	Unable to console, distract or reassure.	
			TOTAL	

Figure 1: Pain Assessment in Advanced Dementia (PAINAD) scale. (Warden et al., 2003)

Dysphagia

Dysphagia is especially common in older adults who live in LTC facilities, with a prevalence of 40% to 50% in this population (Easterling & Robbins, 2008). Disordered swallowing can arise from a number of factors, including motor, sensory, or behavioural factors (Easterling & Robbins, 2008), all of which can occur in dementia. In dementia, the presence of dysphagia can lead to dehydration, aspiration pneumonia, malnutrition, and weight loss (Easterling & Robbins, 2008). Symptoms of dysphagia include coughing, throat clearing, and voice quality changes. Clinical bedside screening performed by a physician can be used to assess the signs of dysphagia (Easterling & Robbins, 2008).

It has been found that patients with dementia who required feeding or cuing at mealtime were at greater risk of mortality and concurrent illness than patients who can feed themselves (Easterling & Robbins, 2008). Thus, it is important to establish proper feeding techniques and educate patients and their caregivers on safe swallowing strategies in attempt to prevent aspiration events and dehydration, and minimize weight loss (Easterling & Robbins, 2008). A speech language pathologist and dietician can work in conjunction with the patient and family to devise a plan to ensure safe swallowing and meet dietary needs. Altering the patient's posture as well as modifying the bolus volume and consistency are some of the techniques to consider (Easterling & Robbins, 2008). Other strategies such as eliminating distractions, a consistent mealtime routine, and providing several small meals during the day are also used to support proper feeding and hydration (Easterling & Robbins, 2008). In the presented case study, Mrs. A was seen by both a speech language pathologist and dietician for creation of an optimal meal plan to minimize choking hazards and maximize nutrition.

Dyspnea

Dyspnea has been seen to be poorly managed in patients with dementia (Sternberg et al., 2014). Pneumonia is the main cause, but it can also be secondary to pulmonary edema (Arcand, 2015). Opioids are the most effective treatment for dyspnea management at the end of life. Other medications such as loop diuretics (ie. furosemide), benzodiazepines (ie. midazolam), and supplemental oxygen (Arcand, 2015) may be used to relieve discomfort. Side effects of these drugs should not be underestimated and kept in mind, with regular risk and benefit discussions as needs arise. Dyspnea can also evoke fear and anxiety in family members, and education about the expected changes in breathing patterns at the end of life should be communicated in a timely manner to minimize frustration.

Cachexia

Cachexia is a complex metabolic process that involves anorexia and severe wasting, particularly loss of fat and muscle mass (Minaglia et al., 2019). It is a condition often associated with terminal illnesses, including advanced dementia. This is thought to be due to the interplay between sarcopenia, malnutrition, and inactivity, which are all of increased prevalence with aging (Minaglia et al., 2019). As cachexia increases morbidity and mortality, it is condition of high clinical relevance (Minaglia et al., 2019). Cachexia contributes to frailty and overall failure to thrive in patients with dementia.

Anorexia is the loss of appetite and decreased intake of food observed frequently with aging later in life. Anorexia is a main characteristic of cachexia (Minaglia et al., 2019) leading to early satiety, due to alteration in fundal compliance, increase in antral stretch and cholecystokinin activity (Minaglia et al., 2019). Sarcopenia is associated with loss of skeletal muscle mass, which is another main characteristic of cachexia. Approximately 50% of older adults over the age of 80 are affected by sarcopenia (Minaglia et al., 2019). It is also of high concern in those suffering from dementia as it associated with risk of falls, poor quality of life, and increased mortality (Minaglia et al., 2019).

Frailty

Frailty has been associated with dementia (Borges et al., 2019; M. Li et al., 2020; C. Wang et al., 2017). Frail individuals have been seen to have a higher risk of dementia compared to non-frail individuals (Borges et al.,

2019; M. Li et al., 2020). Frailty is defined as a state of increased vulnerability to stressors resulting in age-related changes. It is a pathological aging process that has a prevalence of 10% in the geriatric population (Borges et al., 2019). In primary care, frailty is diagnosed via Fried's frailty phenotype (consisting of slow walking speed, impaired grip strength, declining levels of physical activity, exhaustion, and unintentional weight loss), and/or the frailty index, which examines health deficits (Won, 2020). Frailty can be managed through adequate physical activity, addressing nutrition, oral health, and social support (Won, 2020). Frailty may be a risk factor for dementia (Borges et al., 2019). The frailty index may assist healthcare providers in identifying older adults who may be at risk of dementia (C. Wang et al., 2017). Gaining further understanding on the link between frailty and cognitive impairment in the older population may assist with the development of strategies to manage both issues (Borges et al., 2019). The Karnofsky Performance Scale (KPS) (Figure 2) assesses severity of weight loss, fatigue, and difficulty with self-care and daily activities (Continua Hospice Learning, n.d.). The Palliative Performance Scale (PPS) (Figure 3) (Visiting Nurse Service of New York, n.d.) is a modification of the KPS (Anderson et al., 1996), which can also be used to assess frailty in dementia patients.

KARNOFSKY PERFORMANCE STATUS SCALE DEFINITIONS RATING (%) CRITERIA

Able to carry on normal activity and to work; no special care needed.	100	Normal no complaints; no evidence of disease.
	90	Able to carry on normal activity; minor signs or symptoms of disease.
	80	Normal activity with effort; some signs or symptoms of disease.
Unable to work; able to live at home and care for most personal needs; varying amount of assistance needed.	70	Cares for self; unable to carry on normal activity or to do active work.
	60	Requires occasional assistance, but is able to care for most of his personal needs.
	50	Requires considerable assistance and frequent medical care.
Unable to care for self; requires equivalent of institutional or hospital care; disease may be progressing rapidly.	40	Disable; requires special care and assistance.
	30	Severely disabled; hospital admission is indicated although death not imminent.
	20	Very sick; hospital admission necessary; active supportive treatment necessary.
	10	Moribund; fatal processes progressing rapidly.
	0	Dead

Figure 2: Karnofsky Performance Scale (Continua Hospice Learning)

Palliative Performance Scale (PPSv2) version 2[2]

PPS Level	Ambulation	Activity & Evidence of Disease	Self-Care	Intake	Conscious Level
100%	Full	Normal activity & work / No evidence of disease	Full	Normal	Full
90%	Full	Normal activity & work / Some evidence of disease	Full	Normal	Full
80%	Full	Normal activity with effort / Some evidence of disease	Full	Normal or reduced	Full
70%	Reduced	Unable to do normal job/work / Significant disease	Full	Normal or reduced	Full
60%	Reduced	Unable to do hobby/housework / Significant disease	Occasional assistance necessary	Normal or reduced	Full or confusion
50%	Mainly sit/lie	Unable to do any work / Extensive disease	Considerable assistance required	Normal or reduced	Full or confusion
40%	Mainly in bed	Unable to do most activity / Extensive disease	Mainly assistance	Normal or reduced	Full or drowsy +/- confusion
30%	Totally bed bound	Unable to do any activity / Extensive disease	Total care	Normal or reduced	Full or drowsy +/- confusion
20%	Totally bed bound	Unable to do any activity / Extensive disease	Total care	Minimal to sips	Full or drowsy +/- confusion
10%	Totally bed bound	Unable to do any activity / Extensive disease	Total care	Mouth care only	Drowsy or coma +/- confusion
0%	Death				

Stable: 100%–80%
Hospice Appropriate: 70%–0%

Figure 3: Palliative Performance Scale (Visiting Nurse Service of New York)

Cognitive Impairment

Cognitive impairment in dementia can effectuate frustration and dismay in both the patient and their caregivers. Assessment of cognitive impairment presents many challenges. In order to obtain an accurate evaluation, it is recommended that history is obtained from both the patients and another reliable individual, such as a family member or caregiver (Hugo & Ganguli, 2014). Objective assessment tools can also be utilized, which require one or more standardized tests. Examples include the Mini-Mental State Examination (MMSE) and the Montreal Cognitive Assessment (MoCA) (Hugo & Ganguli, 2014). It has been shown that treatment with cholinesterase inhibitors (ie. donepezil, rivastigmine, and galantamine) has yielded modest improvements in cognitive function and everyday activities in patients with Alzheimer's disease. Galantamine has been seen to be effective as a first line therapy for neuropsychiatric symptoms in dementia, while risperidone is more effective when symptoms of agitation and irritability are present (Freund-Levi et al., 2014), and Mrs. A's case could be a good example. However, the side effects of this group of medications should be considered and the awareness of possible induction of agitation should be widespread between health care professionals. For example, donepezil has been seen to be associated with the onset of mania (Leung, 2014), as well as gastrointestinal side effects such as nausea and vomiting (Jackson et al., 2004). Galantamine and rivastigmine may also lead to gastrointestinal side effects resulting in abdominal pain (Mimica & Presecki, 2009). Cognitive enhancers can also have cardiac side effects including bradycardia, rhythm abnormalities, and heart block (Mimica & Presecki, 2009), leading to repeated falls. Other potential pharmacologic agents include N-methyl-D-aspartate (NMDA) receptor antagonists, serotonergic agents, dopamine blocking agents, and benzodiazepines (Hugo & Ganguli, 2014). These medications should be discontinued in a timely manner as the illness progresses and no benefit is expected anymore to minimize the burden associated with medication intake and side effects. Education of healthcare professionals including primary care providers and specialists, as well as the public, is required. This will create awareness in order to mitigate resistance associated with withdrawing these medications when no benefit from them can be expected anymore, or side effects are causing more discomfort, especially when this population is approaching end of life.

Anxiety

Anxiety is a common symptom in the dementia population, affecting up to 71% of patients (Kwak et al., 2017). This symptom significantly reduces quality of life. Anxiety is difficult to diagnose and quantify, and the differentiation of anxiety from other neuropsychiatric symptoms in dementia can present challenges (Kwak et al., 2017). There is little agreement on the guidelines to define anxiety in the dementia setting, and the impaired communication in this disease muddles this assessment more (Kwak et al., 2017). Behavioural interventions such as cognitive behavioural therapy have been seen to be beneficial (Kwak et al., 2017). Pharmacologic therapies such as anxiolytics, antidepressants, cholinesterase inhibitors, and antipsychotics can also be used (Kwak et al., 2017), but not without limitations and side effects should be considered following risk-benefit assessment prior to prescribing. Non-pharmacological management of anxiety associated with responsive behaviour of dementia is preferable. Therapeutic touch therapy has been seen to be safe and well-tolerated in a geriatric PC setting, and was successful as a supportive therapy in aiding patients to achieve a state of relaxation and sleep as well as supporting caregivers (Senderovich et al., 2016).

Responsive Behaviours

Responsive behaviours, such as aggression, agitation, and restlessness, can occur in dementia patients for various reasons (Alzheimer

Society of Canada, 2019). As dementia is a neurological disorder, changes in behaviour may occur as the disease progresses (Alzheimer Society of Canada, 2019). Responsive behaviours may be a result of neurological damage, inability or difficulty to communicate, frustration, confusion, depression, delirium, and/or pain (Alzheimer Society of Canada, 2019). These behaviours, especially if resistant to treatment, can create challenges in the management of dementia. In order to address and manage these behaviours, it is important to understand the root of them (ie. physical discomfort, social isolation, lack of human contact), and accordingly adjust environmental stimuli for the patient (Alzheimer Society of Canada, 2019). Depending on the situation, shifting the patient's focus from these behaviours may also be useful. Non-pharmacological approaches, such as therapeutic touch, have been shown to be beneficial for managing responsive behaviours in patients with dementia, to target restlessness and vocalization, as well as promote states of relaxation, with no negative sequelae (Senderovich et al., 2016; Woods et al., 2005).

Palliative Continuous Deep Sedation and Medical Assistance in Dying

Continuous deep sedation (CDS) may be a viable treatment option for patients with dementia when symptoms become unmanageable and/or there is no response to disease modifying therapy, resulting in suffering and poor quality of the remaining life. CDS may be within the goals of care for some patients and should be discussed at the time of ACP. CDS utilizes medications to induce an unconscious state in order to relieve suffering and control refractory symptoms (Bravo et al., 2018), such as pain, dyspnea, and neuropsychiatric symptoms, including agitation, anxiety, and symptoms of terminal delirium. This is usually done when life expectancy is two weeks or less (Bravo et al., 2018). CDS has not been associated with decreased survival or acceleration of death (Schur et al., 2016; Yokomichi et al., 2022).

Medical assistance in dying (MAiD) was legalized in Canada in 2016 for patients with a life-limiting illness that met the legal requirements (Bravo et al., 2018). Previously, dementia patients in Canada were not eligible for MAiD, as it was required that the patient remains competent to give final consent at the time of the procedure. This requirement was waived, and it is now required for the patient to be competent at the time they request MAiD while partaking in ACP during earlier stages of the illness, however some clinicians may interpret this eligibility characteristic as unmet. In order to qualify for MAiD, individuals must be experiencing an advanced state of decline that cannot be reversed (Pope, 2021). There are still multiple obstacles for dementia patients to receive MAiD and most of them are related to withdrawal of final consent, which involves the requirement for foreseeable death, incapacitated vetoes (in the case when the patient seems to indicate that they no longer want MAiD once they have lost decision-making capacity), and unwillingness from clinicians (Pope, 2021). Overall, studies showed that Canadian physicians seemed to support offering MAiD to incompetent end-stage patients with dementia if advance requests were made (Bravo et al., 2018; Nakanishi et al., 2021).

CDS can be compared and contrasted to MAiD. CDS and MAiD are similar in the sense that they respect patient autonomy and alleviate suffering (Booker & Bruce, 2020). Differences include theoretical reversibility (in the case of CDS), prognosis (where CDS is administered at a life expectancy of two weeks or less, and MAiD when death is "reasonably foreseeable"), and public awareness (the degree of public awareness is higher for MAiD, especially due to media exposure) (Booker & Bruce, 2020). Additionally, CDS can be titrated to the desired state and thus administered in a proportional manner [ie. to achieve a score of (-1) to (-5) on the Richmond Agitation-Sedation Scale (RASS), according to the Alberta Health Services guideline for palliative sedation] and based on goals of care (Booker & Bruce, 2020). The RASS range of scores of (-5) to (+4) is used to classify different levels of agitation and sedation, with scores of (-5) to (-1) being used to classify sedation [with (-5) being the highest level of sedation (unarousable) and (-1) being the lightest level of sedation (drowsy, not completely alert)], and scores of (+1) to (+4) being used to classify agitation [with (+4) being the highest level of agitation]. CDS differs from MAiD in this sense, as MAiD can be viewed as disproportionate and having an "all or nothing" approach.

Deprescribing in Dementia

Polypharmacy, defined as the use of multiple medications by a patient simultaneously, is often observed in older population. Many of these medications may also have detrimental side effects. In dementia, where quality of life and comfort are of high priority, risk-benefit analyses may determine whether it is beneficial to terminate the use of certain medications in order to improve the quality of the remaining life. PC consultation and timely integration of PC may be useful in patients' management. In the setting of a life-limiting illness, the division between life-extending, complication-preventing management and symptomatic therapy remains unclear (Abel, 2013). It is a gradual process and should be evaluated on an individual basis (Abel, 2013), and based on goals of care. The need for medications also lessens at the end of life, due to metabolism changes in the body and the lack of benefit (Abel, 2013). It is also important to consider which stage the patient is at in their illness, and the extent to which the patient and their family have accepted mortality (Abel, 2013). ACP also plays a role in allowing a comfortable transition from life-extending interventions to symptomatic therapy, to benefit both the patient and the family (Abel, 2013). In the presented case study, near the end of life Mrs. A's healthcare team deprescribed various of her long-term medications, including statins, antihypertensives, and multivitamins to minimize pill burden.

Benefits of Deprescribing

Patients with end-stage dementia are often taking numerous medications. However, not all of these medications may be appropriate or deemed to be suitable with a proper risk-benefit analysis. A chart review study conducted by Holmes et al. (2008) examined the medication use in patients with advanced dementia (Holmes et al., 2008). It was determined that 5% of prescribed medications were never appropriate (according to the Delphi consensus panel), and 29% of patients had been on a never appropriate medication (Holmes et al., 2008). Pype et al. (2017) found a high level of use of potentially inappropriate medications in primary care at the end of life (Pype et al., 2018). The practice of deprescribing inappropriate medications, especially in the end stages of life, would minimize unpleasant side effects and ultimately improve the quality of life for dementia patients.

Deprescribing comes hand in hand with reduced pharmacy costs and healthcare saving (Reeve et al., 2014). Araw et al. (2015) performed a retrospective study involving end-stage dementia patients, where they found that after PC consultation, there was a significant reduction in daily pharmacy cost (Araw et al., 2015). Patients were also provided with appropriate medications to meet their needs, control symptoms, and improve quality of life, including analgesics and anti-emetics. A randomized controlled trial by Curtin et al. (2020) found that deprescribing led to a reduction in polypharmacy and medication costs in frail older patients (Curtin et al., 2020). Deprescribing results in reversal of the effects of polypharmacy and leads to positive clinical outcomes (Garfinkel, 2018). Prioritizing symptom relief management leads to cost reduction and healthcare saving.

Appropriate Medication to Deprescribe
Cognitive Enhancer Medications

Cognitive enhancers are often used in dementia for the prevention of further memory decline, and controlling behavioural issues. Cholinesterase inhibitors and memantine are the main drugs in this class. Discontinuing these medications at the end of life may help to minimize adverse drug reactions and pill burden, and as a result improve the quality of life in dementia patients (Reeve et al., 2019). There is evidence of a small but significant risk of bradycardia and syncope with the use of anticholinesterase inhibitors (Howes, 2014), which frequently leads to falls and associated injury. The benefits and harms of these medications can shift over time with long-term use (Reeve et al., 2019), which renders them an appropriate candidate for deprescribing especially at the end of life when no further benefit is expected from these drugs.

Deprescribing of cognitive enhancers should be done through shared decision making between the patients who preserved their capacity to participate in this process and caregivers (Reeve et al., 2019). It is beneficial to have a discussion outlining goals of treatment and a cost-benefit of these drugs at the beginning of therapy and continue revisiting this throughout the illness trajectory (Reeve et al., 2019). Communication with caregivers outlining the illness trajectory and expected cognitive decline with the progression of the disease is crucial (Reeve et al., 2019). If required, other medications can be used for comfort and controlling behavioural issues.

Neuroleptics

Neuroleptics are a first-line therapy for the treatment of neuropsychiatric symptoms. In dementia, these symptoms may include agitation, aggression, and psychosis (Ballard et al., 2008). However, there are concerns regarding the safety of long-term use of neuroleptics in dementia and the risks associated with stroke, sedation, edema, chest infection, and worsening of cognitive decline (Ballard et al., 2008). Extrapyramidal symptoms such as parkinsonism can also lead to falls and decreased mobility. A randomized, blinded, placebo-controlled trial by Ballard et al. (2008) revealed that the discontinuation of neuroleptics did not present detrimental effects on cognitive and functional status (Ballard et al., 2008). Results portray that there is not a benefit of continuing this treatment in patients with dementia, and neuroleptics should not be used as first-line therapy (Ballard et al., 2008). Neuroleptics should also be withdrawn at the end of life to maximize quality of life. The search for a better solution for neuropsychiatric symptoms in dementia is strongly encouraged (Ballard et al., 2008). Nonpharmacological interventions such as music therapy, touch therapy, and activity programs showed positive effects in dementia patients and can be utilized as adjuvants (de Oliveira et al., 2015).

Antihypertensive Medications

Antihypertensive medications are commonly used in older adults to control blood pressure. However, in terminally ill patients, low blood pressure is observed frequently, and thus antihypertensives should be discontinued (Parsons et al., 2010). Hypotension can result in dizziness and lead to repeated falls, fractures and other injuries. Weight loss associated with cachexia may also permit the withdrawal of these drugs (Parsons et al., 2010). Ekbom et al. (1994) found that the discontinuation of antihypertensive medications in older patients can be attempted without the increased risk of cardiovascular events, with the implementation of regular monitoring (Ekbom et al., 1994). Interestingly, there is also a shift in the relationship between blood pressure and mortality in individuals that are 85 years or older, where low systolic blood pressure contributed to a higher mortality rate (Harrison et al., 2016).

Vitamins and Supplements

Vitamins and supplements are utilized for the management of fatigue and metabolic imbalance. However, at the end of life they become non-essential based on the goals of care and should be withdrawn to minimize pill burden, medication side effects such as hypervitaminosis, electrolyte imbalance, potential interaction with essential medications (Whitman et al., 2018) and other complications, especially in the absence of monitoring of blood parameters.

Comparison of Deprescribing in Practice

Physicians' views on deprescribing in older patients are variable across medical specialties. While there may be a range of perspectives, the common goal is to decrease polypharmacy, pill burden, and adverse drug reactions. A study exploring deprescribing practices of general practitioners

(GPs) in frail older patients revealed that GPs deprescribing was based on impact to quality of life, patient's wishes, risk and benefit analysis of medications, and life expectancy (Mantelli et al., 2018). There was also inclination to deprescribe cardiovascular medication in both patients with and without cardiovascular disease, while retaining pain medication (Mantelli et al., 2018). Dolara (2020) discussed the challenges associated with deprescribing in the setting of clinical cardiology, noting that adverse effects of withdrawal pose an obstacle (Dolara, 2020). However, in certain settings such as advanced dementia, withdrawing certain medications such as statins would be appropriate (Dolara, 2020), especially in the setting of limited life expectancy. It is recommended that collaboration be established between cardiologists, who initially prescribe medications, and GPs who follow patients long-term (Dolara, 2020). A study comparing the deprescribing practices of cardiovascular medications between general internists, geriatricians, and cardiologists revealed that the rationale for deprescribing across all specialties was adverse drug reactions (Goyal et al., 2020). Challenges for deprescribing that were shared across all specialities were concern about interference with the treatment plans of other physicians, as well as hesitancy of patients. Geriatricians reported higher rates of deprescribing in patients with limited life expectancy, and were more likely than other specialties to deprescribe cardiovascular medications in conditions including Alzheimer's disease, recurrent metastatic cancer, and significant functional impairment (Goyal et al., 2020). In the setting of LTC, it was found that obstacles for deprescribing included lack of understanding of indications and harms of stopping the medications by patients and caregivers, time constraints, and collaboration between professionals in the care of the patient (Palagyi et al., 2016). GPs were viewed as crucial to the success of deprescribing initiatives (Palagyi et al., 2016).

    A study assessing factors that influence physician decision-making for deprescribing medications for patients with dementia at the end of life revealed that physicians had some variability regarding the continuation or discontinuation of acetylcholinesterase inhibitors and memantine, and less variability for statins and antipsychotics (Parsons et al., 2014). It has been recommended that there should be development of strategies for PC patients with life-limiting illness, involving discussions about the patient expectations, planning of timely medication withdrawal, and encouraging involvement of various stakeholders in decision making about the patient's management (Todd et al., 2016).

Prognostication

Prognostication is assessment used to guide healthcare professionals in end of life decision making (S. L. Mitchell et al., 2010). Awareness of disease prognosis greatly assists in the ease of end of life care planning. The Gold Standards Framework Proactive Identification Guidance (PIG) is a resource centered around early identification of patients' decline, in order to promote quality care and living and dying well (The Gold Standards Framework, 2022) (Figure 4). This includes patients with any condition, including dementia. In order to identify individuals who are likely to be approaching the end of life, this guideline recommends using a three-step approach (Figure 5), where Step 1 is the "surprise question" (SQ) (Figure 6), Step 2 is general indicators of decline (Figure 7), and Step 3 is specific clinical indicators (The Gold Standards Framework, 2022). The SQ has been found to be a better predictor for death than intuition ($p=0.001$) with a specificity of 80.2% (Downar et al., 2017; G. K. Mitchell et al., 2018) and thus can be utilized as a trigger for timely referral to PC. According to the PIG, dementia-specific clinical indicators that suggest entrance into a later stage of disease include inability to recognize family members, complete dependence on others for care, recurrent delirium, aspiration pneumonia, and urinary and fecal incontinence, in addition to weight loss, urinary tract infections, skin failure, recurrent fever, and reduced oral intake (Figure 8) (The Gold Standards Framework, 2022). The PIG also recommends recognition of moderate or advanced dementia with tools such as the Comprehensive Geriatric Assessment, Clinical Frailty Scale, Functional Assessment Staging, Electronic Frailty Index, or Rockwood Scale (The Gold Standards Framework, 2022).

In addition to the PIG, the KPS, as seen in Figure 2 (Continua Hospice Learning, n.d.), may also be used for prognostication in dementia patients as it reflects on various factors related to loss of function as a result of frailty, which is prevalent in this population (Borges et al., 2019). The PPS (Figure 3) is a valid tool which is often used for assessing physical state and prognostication in dementia patients. Decrease in PPS scores have been shown to be correlated with shorter stays in hospice and time to death (Nasr, 2021).

However, there are limitations to these measures and unfortunately there is not currently an accurate method for determining prognosis in dementia patients. Despite its suitable specificity, the SQ has poor sensitivity (67%) and thus a high rate of false positives (Downar et al., 2017). The high false positive rate may be attributed to various factors, including different opinions among clinicians, reluctance to use the SQ due to clinician discomfort, and reluctance of clinicians to give a positive answer even if they suspect death of the patient (Downar et al., 2017). The SQ is also less accurate in predicting death in noncancerous illness (Downar et al., 2017). The Functional Assessment Staging 7c criterion was also shown to be unreliable in the predication of 6-month mortality in dementia (Brown et al., 2013; Senderovich & Retnasothie, 2020). Although the PPS has demonstrated accuracy when used as a tool for prognostication in cancer, unfortunately it was found unreliable in the setting of dementia as it did not accurately identify patients with medium-term limited life expectancy (Linklater et al., 2011, 2012; Senderovich & Retnasothie, 2020). Overall, despite varying results, the integration of PC early in disease course is critical for quality person-centred care.

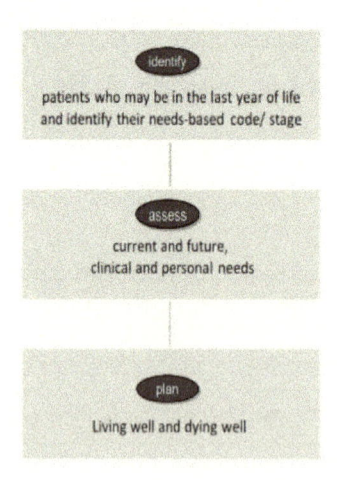

Figure 4: Three Key Steps of the Gold Standards Framework (The Gold Standards Framework, 2022)

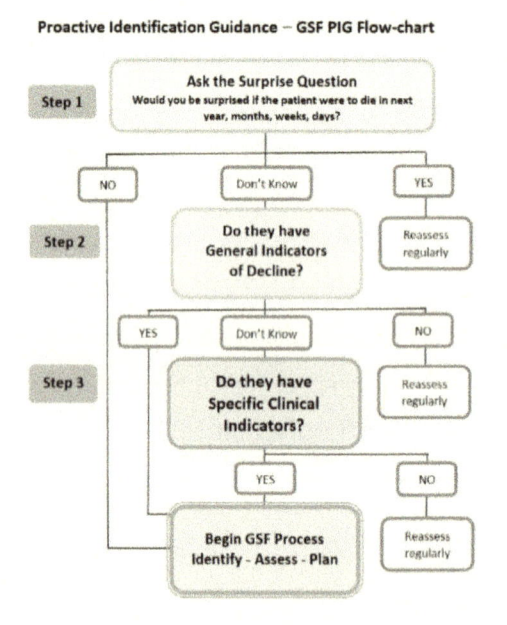

Figure 5: The Gold Standards Framework PIG Flow-Chart (The Gold Standards Framework, 2022)

STEP 1: The Surprise Question
For patients with advanced disease or progressive life limiting conditions, would you be surprised if the patient were to die in the next year, months, weeks, days?
The answer to this question should be an intuitive one, pulling together a range of clinical, social and other factors that give a whole picture of deterioration. If you would not be surprised, then what measures might be taken to improve the patient's quality of life now and in preparation for possible further decline?
This includes proactive planning of care and treatments and offering advance care planning and DNACPR discussions as early as possible.

Figure 6: The Surprise Question (The Gold Standards Framework, 2022)

STEP 2: General indicators of decline and increasing needs
- General physical decline, increasing dependence and need for support
- Repeated unplanned hospital admissions or acute crises at home
- Advanced disease - unstable, deteriorating, complex symptom burden
- Presence of significant multi-morbidities
- Decreasing activity – functional performance status declining (e.g., Barthel or Karnofsky Performance score, Rockwood) limited self-care, in bed or chair 50% of day and increasing dependence in activities of daily living
- Decreasing response to treatments, decreasing reversibility
- Patient choice for no further active treatment, focus on quality of life
- Progressive weight loss (>10%) in past six months
- Sentinel Event e.g., serious fall, carer distress, bereavement, transfer to nursing home, etc
- Serum albumin <25g/l
- Considered eligible for DS1500 payment

Figure 7: The Gold Standards Framework PIG General Indicators of Decline (The Gold Standards Framework, 2022)

DEMENTIA
Identification of moderate/severe stage dementia using a validated tool or Comprehensive Geriatric Assessment (CGA) of frailty, Clinical Frailty Scale (CFS), Functional Assessment Staging, Electronic Frailty Index (EFI) or Rockwood scale, identifying decline in dementia or frailty. Triggers to consider that indicate that someone is entering a later stage are:
- Unable to recognise family members or consistently unable to have meaningful conversations
- Completely dependent on others for care or unable to do ADL
- Recurrent episodes of delirium
- Aspiration pneumonia
- Urinary and faecal incontinence, and Barthel score <3

Plus: Weight loss, urinary tract Infection, skin failure or stage 3 or 4 pressures ulcers, recurrent fever, reduced oral intake

Figure 8: The Gold Standards Framework PIG Dementia-Specific Clinical Indicators (The Gold Standards Framework, 2022)

Models of Palliative Care

As there is currently a lack of formal guidelines for implementation of PC in dementia, there is no current best model. PC in dementia is limitedly systematized, as compared to in cancer treatment (Iliffe et al., 2013). Care at end of life for dementia patients may also be fragmented, with symptoms and pain going unrecognized or untreated (Jones et al., 2016). Overall, there is a need for development of an evidence-based system for provision of high quality PC in dementia globally (Parker, 2021). Two approaches will be discussed below: the COMPASSION Intervention (Jones et al., 2016; Moore et al., 2017) and the IMPACT project (Iliffe et al., 2013).

The COMPASSION Intervention consists of two core components: 1; facilitation of a multidisciplinary approach to assessment, treatment and care, and 2; education, training and support for caregivers (Moore et al., 2017). This model is led by an interdisciplinary care leader, who ensures the intervention scopes local practice, meaning that the intervention complements the existing local practices, and key personnel are supporting end of life care (Moore et al., 2017). The responsibilities of this leader also entail organizing activities structured around the two core components (Moore et al., 2017). Activities for component 1 include person-centred assessment of residents multiple needs to target physical, psychological, social, and emotional domains of care, and engagement of multidisciplinary teams (Moore et al., 2017). Activities for component 2 include training, education and support sessions for staff and family caregivers (Moore et al., 2017).

The IMPACT (Implementation of quality indicators in Palliative Care sTudy) project defined a generic model of PC in Europe, which can be seen in Figure 9. The IMPACT framework consists of active symptom management, focus on the psychosocial needs of patients, and care coordination (Iliffe et al., 2013). This project also posits training and continuous learning of healthcare providers, regular audits of outcomes as a form of learning, stable leadership, and a skill mix among direct healthcare providers to mainstay end of life care (Iliffe et al., 2013). The IMPACT team also is targeting multiple aspects that affect quality of PC in dementia, including: division of labour, responsibilities of providers from different disciplines and its impact on learning, the structure and function of care planning, managing risk and complexity, boundaries between disease-modifying treatment, PC, and bereavement (Iliffe et al., 2013).

The Empowering Better End-of-Life Dementia Care (EMBED-Care) Programme is an example of a novel model of PC specifically for patients with dementia that is currently under research and development. It is based in the United Kingdom and focuses on the development and testing of an intervention that will be designed for patients suffering from dementia, their caregivers, and healthcare providers (Sampson et al., 2020). EMBED-Care is a large collaborative multi-part project with an overall goal of delivering a step change in care for patients affected by dementia, to ensure the best possible care (Sampson et al., 2020). The protocol, as seen in Figure 10, is designed to implement systematic integrated PC in facilities and providing care to patients with dementia at home (Sampson et al., 2020).

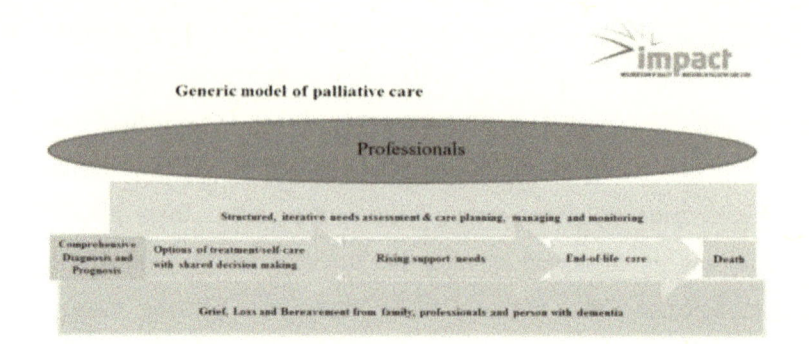

Figure 9: Generic Model of Palliative Care, as defined by the IMPACT project (Iliffe et al., 2013)

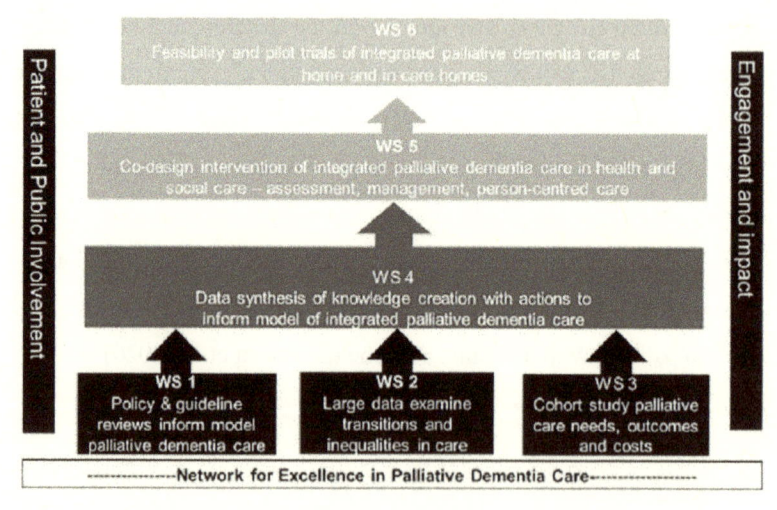

Figure 10: Methods of EMBED-Care Programme (Sampson et al., 2020)

Illness Trajectory and Progress

Dementia is a terminal illness that patients can die with or from (van der Steen et al., 2017). Dementia trajectory is associated with progressive physical disability and decline in cognitive and physical functioning. Patients become frail and emaciated, and may experience death from an acute event (ie. a fracture) (Murray et al., 2005). A graphical representation of the trajectory of dementia (falling in the category of physical and cognitive frailty), in comparison to the trajectories of cancer and organ failure, is depicted in Figure 11 (Murray & Sheikh, 2008). As can be seen in Figure 11, out of trajectory categories shown, the category of physical and cognitive frailty had the greatest amount of deaths. Overall, understanding disease trajectory may assist healthcare providers in planning goals of care and help to create a care plan to maximize quality of life and dignified death for those affected by this illness.

A commonly used scale for rating of the various stages of dementia is the Global Deterioration Scale for Assessment of Primary Degenerative Dementia (GDS), also known as the Reisberg Scale. This scale classifies dementia based on the level of cognitive decline, and includes seven stages, which are described in Table 1 (Reisberg et al., 1982). This scale has been successfully validated against behavioural, neuroanatomic, and neurophysiologic measures in dementia patients (Reisberg et al., 1982).

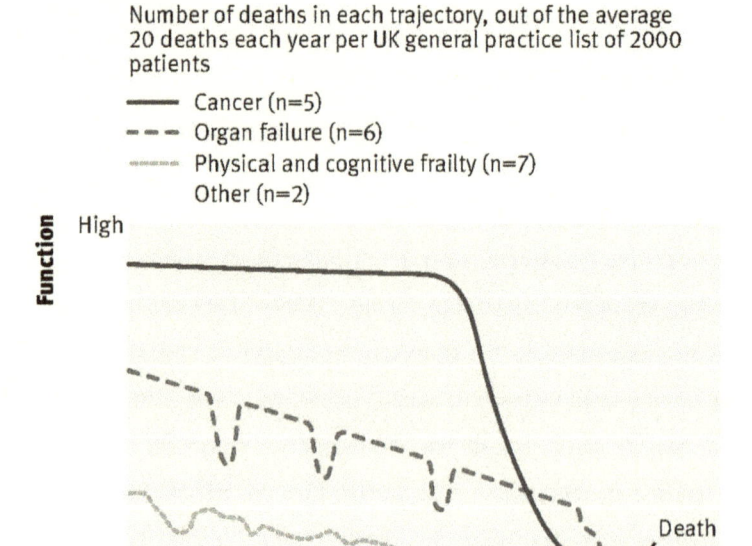

Number of deaths in each trajectory, out of the average 20 deaths each year per UK general practice list of 2000 patients

— Cancer (n=5)
--- Organ failure (n=6)
⋯ Physical and cognitive frailty (n=7)
Other (n=2)

Figure 11: Disease trajectory of illnesses at the end of life (Murray & Sheikh, 2008).

Table 1: GDS/Reisberg Scale for Assessment of Stages of Dementia (Reisberg et al., 1982).

DIAGNOSIS	STAGE	SIGNS AND SYMPTOMS	AVERAGE DURATION
No Dementia	Stage 1: No Cognitive Decline	• Normal function and no loss of memory	N/A
No Dementia	Stage 2: Very Mild Cognitive Decline	• Forgets names and misplaces objects • Symptoms not clear to healthcare providers or family/friends	Unknown
No Dementia	Stage 3: Mild Cognitive Decline	• Forgetfulness increasing • Anomic aphasia	2 to 7 years

		• Beginning to have difficulty with concentration • Symptoms start to become evident to family/friends	
Early Dementia	Stage 4: Moderate Cognitive Decline	• Forgets recent events • Difficulty with concentration • Difficulty with task completion • Social withdrawal • Denial • Symptoms evident to healthcare providers	2 years
Mid-Stage Dementia	Stage 5: Moderately Severe Cognitive Decline	• Significant memory issues • Requires assistance with daily living tasks • Loss of awareness of time, date, and location	1.5 years
Mid-Stage Dementia	Stage 6: Severe Cognitive Decline	• Forgets recent events and major past events • Forgets name of family members • Difficulty with speaking • Cannot carry out daily living tasks without help • Changes in emotions and personality • Anxiety • Delusions • Incontinence	2.5 years
Late Dementia	Stage 7: Very Severe Cognitive Decline	• Loss of speech/communication • Loss of motor skills • Loss of mobility	1.5 to 2.5 years

NOTE: Dysphagia (not listed here) can prevail in earlier stages, and progress with disease duration (Payne & Morley, 2018).

Benefits of Palliative Care

The integration of PC in dementia has the potential to yield multiple benefits. These advantages have a large span and affect patients, caregivers, and the healthcare system.

Quality of Life and Comfort

As mentioned previously, dementia has a wide array of physical, cognitive, and emotional symptoms. As the end of life nears, symptom management becomes increasingly pronounced (Hendriks et al., 2017). PC would allow integration of a specialized healthcare team, which is individualized for the specific needs of the patient. This would help to address medical issues that patients may face and ensure that pain and discomfort are properly managed. eHealth interventions may even be utilized, to involve remote specialist input on care (Gillam et al., 2021). Pain in dementia has frequently been related to depression (Gruber-Baldini et al., 2005), therefore adequate pain management will also lead to a lower rate of depression and decreased agitation. It has been speculated that agitation in dementia patients can be associated with pain (Husebo et al., 2014). Lastly, timely consideration of ACP will lead to fulfilling patient wishes and expectations. Thorough recognition and timely management of a patient's symptoms, while simultaneously addressing patient's needs, will lead to the best quality of life of those living with dementia (Harris, 2007).

Reduced Emergency Room Visits

It was found that dementia patients receiving community-based PC had significantly less emergency room visits compared to patients who were not receiving PC (Rosenwax et al., 2015). The reviewed literature showed that most frequently, patients presented to the emergency department with dyspnea, altered consciousness, nausea and vomiting (Rosenwax et al., 2015). Towards the end of life, the frequency of unplanned hospital admissions increased in patients with dementia (Yorganci et al., 2021) as a result of a heightened need for symptom control, which could be reduced through addressing ACP in a timely manner. Repeated hospital readmissions and emergency room visits are not only taxing and stressful for the patient and family, but also burdensome to the healthcare system and incur high costs (Luengo-Fernandez et al., 2011). The timely integration of PC in dementia management can play a role in alleviating this stressor for all parties, leading to the improvement of the quality of remaining life. Adequate symptom control and prevention of repeated emergency room visits leads to improvement of quality of life of patients and their caregivers, and significant healthcare saving.

Good Death

Steinhauser et al. (2000) have outlined six themes for the definition of a good death (Steinhauser et al., 2000). These include: management of pain and symptoms, clear decision making, death preparation, completion of life, contribution to the well-being others, and affirmation of the patient as a whole person (Steinhauser et al., 2000). With the implementation of PC in dementia, measures can be put in place to fulfill these criteria. As patient comfort is a cornerstone of PC, pain and symptom management can be properly addressed by the healthcare team. Additionally, ACP can be explored in a timely manner and a clear decision can be made while the patient is approaching the end stages of life to ensure death will be managed accordingly based on patient's wishes. Through the patient-centred approach that is central to PC, themes outlined by Steinhauser et al. (2000) such as completion, contributing to others, and affirmation of the whole person can be incorporated into care leading to a good death for the patient.

Decreased Stress for Family and Caregivers

Dementia is not only a taxing illness for the patient, but can also cause extreme stress for family and caregivers, ultimately leading to caregiver burden, pressure to make decisions, and worry for the well-being of the patient. A systematic review on PC in dementia management found that families often believed that symptoms were poorly managed in dementia patients (Senderovich & Retnasothie, 2020). This may be associated with a degree of stress and guilt, which could be relieved with proper symptom management. It is also noted that there is an increase of emotional stress associated with caring for patients with dementia, and caregivers are frequently suffering from pre-death grief (Crawley et al., 2021).

Timely integrated PC may support caregivers by offering services and assisting with stress reduction. This may be in the form of education on the patient's illness, bereavement support, or other physical forms of support. Interestingly, the Hospice Caregiver Support Project showed a significant impact on caregivers by reducing stress through helping with care of the patients and assisting with activities of daily living, including providing home delivered meals and aiding with housekeeping duties (Empeño et al., 2011). Social worker support can also benefit both the patient and the family, minimize burden and loss, and improve quality of life and well-being for all parties involved (McGovern, 2015).

Benefits of PC in Dementia

Patient
- Increased quality of life
- Symptom management
- Comfort
- Good death

Family/Caregiver
- Decreased stress
- Decreased guilt
- Reduced caregiver burden

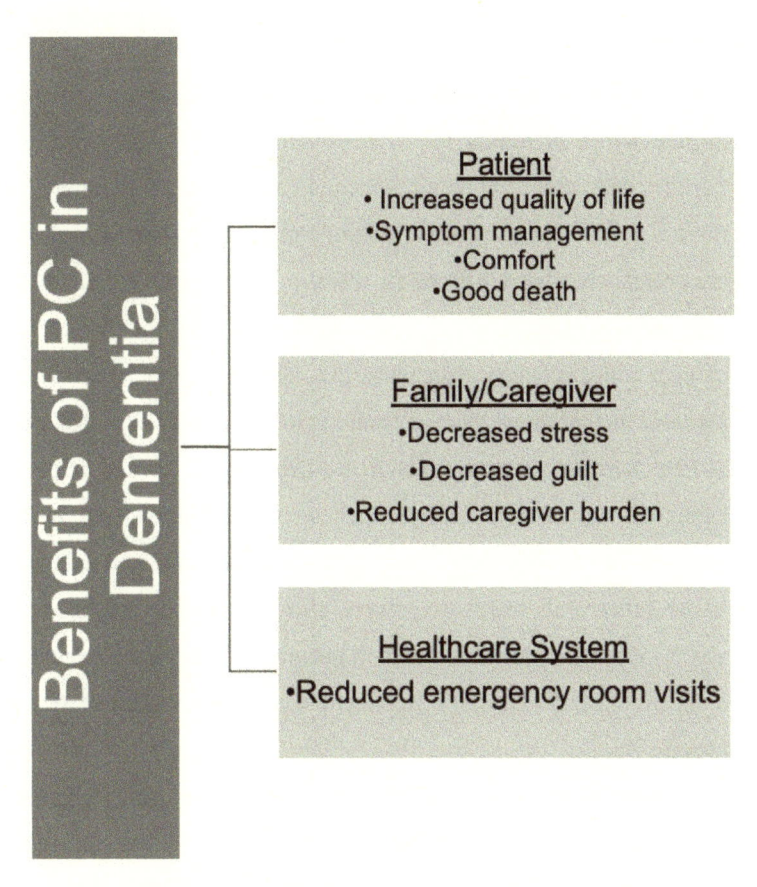

Healthcare System
- Reduced emergency room visits

Figure 12: The Benefits of Palliative Care in Dementia

Recommendations for Palliative Care

Education for patients, families, and caregivers is of paramount importance in providing PC to those suffering from dementia. Teaching families and caregivers about dementia can help the community, however there is a deficit in the amount of family members of dementia patients who are adequately educated about the disease (Pandpazir & Tajari, 2019). It has also been suggested that caregivers should undergo training on providing care to those affected with dementia. This can help to minimize futile invasive interventions, such as feeding tube placement (Pandpazir & Tajari, 2019), increase awareness about the benefits of PC and importance of symptom control, and outline challenges with oral intake in dementia patients. This can also serve provide education on safe swallowing strategies to be utilized in order to prevent choking episode and complications associated with it, such as aspiration pneumonia. Therefore, beginning at the level of the community, it is recommended that sufficient awareness is raised.

Education will also establish a framework for timely PC consultation. Early integration of PC is recommended, based on the National Institute for Health and Clinical Excellence (Harris, 2007) guidelines in the management of dementia. Care for dementia patients should include PC. PC service should be available to dementia patients in the same way it is available to other patients (Harris, 2007). ACP guided by the patient and caregiver is highly important and should be in place (Harris, 2007). It will help to establish goals of care, create a plan for care, and discuss end of life care. NICE guidelines also address the role of the Mental Capacity Act 2005, which relates to decisions made in advance to forgo treatment and select preferred place of care (Harris, 2007). While the patient still maintains the cognitive ability to make these decisions, it is pertinent to initiate discussion surrounding key issues earlier in disease trajectory to ensure that the patient's individual wishes are granted. A main pillar of PC is a patient-centred approach, and treatment should be tailored to unique patient needs and symptom management.

NICE also recommends that when patients with dementia exhibit unexplained behavioural shifts, pain should be ruled out and adequate assessment should take place (Harris, 2007). Approximately 50% of dementia patients experience pain (Achterberg et al., 2013), and this often goes undertreated (Sarbacker, 2014). Therefore, it would be beneficial to monitor the patient carefully to ensure adequate pain control and comfort of the patients. PAINAID is a pain assessment tool that can be utilized in this setting.

Lastly, minimizing inappropriate treatments, such as artificial feeding, is also recommended while caring for dementia patients (Harris, 2007) in order to avoid unnecessary pain, agitation and symptom burden, especially at the point where no quality of life can be expected and the patient is nearing the end of life. Deprescribing medications at the end of life is vital to minimize pill burden and medication related side effects, improve the quality of the remaining life, and decrease pharmacy costs (Araw et al., 2015).

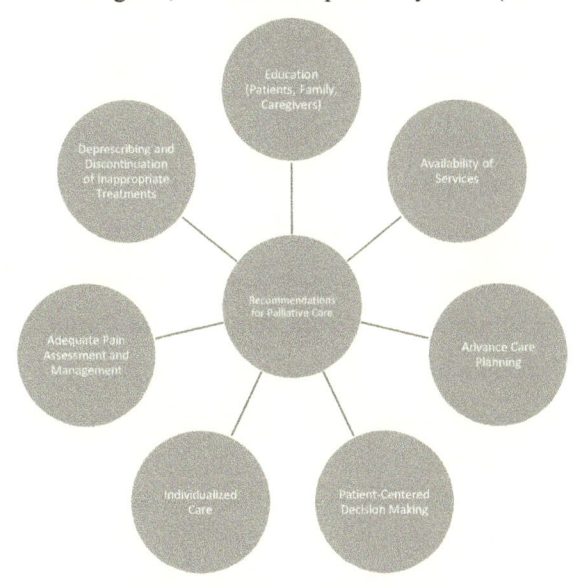

Figure 13: Recommendations for Palliative Care in Dementia

Resource Availability

The resources available for the care of those living with dementia are overall scarce and limited, which raises challenges for the adequate provision of PC to this population at the end-of-life. The majority of older people express that the home is their preferred setting for death, however most will die in the hospital or nursing home setting (Canadian Institute for Health Information, n.d.). In Canada, 67% of acute care patients with dementia were identified as having PC needs (Canadian Institute for Health Information, n.d.), and globally the number of dementia patients who have PC needs is expected to increase by four times over the next 40 years (Sampson et al., 2020). This is problematic as hospital and nursing home staff often have limited training in PC, and more resources are required in this area (Canadian Institute for Health Information, n.d.).

In Canada specifically, LTC homes are lacking resources to provide the highest quality of PC for dementia patients (Hill et al., 2018). A study by Hill et al. discussed multiple resource shortages including funding personnel and supplies (Hill et al., 2018). In the context of dementia, PC is more time-consuming due to communication difficulties and challenges associated with assessment of needs, as well as the requirement to provide a calming environment and reassurance to the patient (Hill et al., 2018), often with the use of supportive counselling. Care is often task-oriented for the sake of time efficiency, which does not align with the patient-centred approach that is a mainstay of PC. Funding limitations impact psychosocial care needs, provided by social workers, chaplains, and recreation therapists and affect adequate staff training in PC for those who are deficient in it (Hill et al., 2018). Overall, little is known about the efforts to address PC barriers in Canada (Hill et al., 2018).

Age-Related Inequalities and Accessibility

Age-related inequalities have persistently affected older persons' accessibility to healthcare. Older age has also been cited as a barrier to PC because practitioners may perceive that death in an older person is not as jarring and that older patients may accept terminal diagnoses more easily (Gardiner et al., 2011). Therefore, there may be a preconceived notion that older patients are less deserving of PC as death is expected. In Canada, age has been shown to be a main predictor of access to PC programs for cancer patients, where older patients has less access, even after controlling for demographic, health service and ecologic variables (Burge et al., 2008). Lindskog et al. (2015) have demonstrated that old age is a risk factor for poor quality of end of life care (Lindskog et al., 2015). These inequalities are also applicable in the setting of PC and dementia, which often affects older population. For this population, there may be challenges with access to healthcare thus affecting quality of life and end of life care. As a matter of fact, a reduction in access to healthcare typically exists for the oldest-old (Cooper et al., 2016). Additionally, socio-economic factors may play a role in accessibility. Decreased physical health and low levels of education are linked to a greater dementia risk (Bullain et al., 2013; Sharp & Gatz, 2011). Older people and women from areas of deprivation are less likely to receive anti-dementia drugs, specifically acetylcholinesterase inhibitors (Cooper et al., 2016), which may represent the inequitable access to healthcare resources in these populations. A population-based register study showed that patients dying from Alzheimer's and dementia had lower quality care at the end of life than patients dying from cancer, which cannot be explained by end of life care guidelines (Martinsson et al., 2018). Mitigation of these barriers is essential for ensuring accessibility to PC for older patients with dementia.

Health System Implications

Although PC provides benefits to the patient, family members, and caregivers, the implications and effects on the health system as a whole must also be considered. Chu et al.'s study found that PC for patients with dementia who resided in LTC facilities had multiple greater benefits (Chu et al., 2020). When utilization of medical services by dementia patients was compared before and after PC, it was found that usage of resources was significantly reduced, including quantity of medical departments visited, quantity of prescribed medications, frequency of hospitalization, and emergency room visits (Chu et al., 2020). Additionally, when examining the quantity of hospital admissions before and after hospice care in patients who died within 6 months after PC program integration, it was found that there was a slight but not significant ($p=0.058$) increase in admission before the integration of the PC program on univariate analysis (Chu et al., 2020). The overall decrease in use of medical services for dementia patients upon the integration of PC is also associated with reductions in cost and burden to the healthcare system. Hospital-based PC units reduced hospital costs by $7000 to $8000 per patient (Batzlaff et al., 2014). Timely integration of PC leads to better symptom control, and can prevent emergency room overcrowding.

There are also barriers and limitations that come with the integration of PC in dementia. Shortages in staffing and physical resources, as well as funding, lead to challenges in providing quality PC and overall stress to the healthcare system. Potential reworking of the logistical structure to overcome these barriers should be considered.

Knowledge Translation

Knowledge translation (KT), a process of disseminating important information to improve healthcare delivery, can be beneficial to healthcare providers, the healthcare system, caregivers, patients, and family members who play a role in patients' management of dementia. Thus education of healthcare professionals and the public is crucial. A narrative review by Phillipson et al. (2016) revealed that multimodal learning strategies were most useful for healthcare providers, and should be applied to the workplace as a whole, as opposed to individuals (Phillipson et al., 2016). Bridging the gap between research and practice also would be beneficial for learners (Phillipson et al., 2016). A cluster randomized controlled trial on the evaluation of a nurse-led program on dementia and knowledge translation in primary care yielded positive impacts on the approach to care for patients with dementia and practice of healthcare professionals (Y. Wang et al., 2017). It has also been found that integrated KT strategies have allowed family caregivers to provide better care to dementia patients in the home setting, by increasing access to support and information for dementia care (Forbes, 2018).

There are also various lessons to be learned about the benefits of integration of end of life care in dementia. Primarily, the introduction of PC early in disease trajectory is imperative. ACP is crucial and should be addressed at the time of diagnosis, as patients often lose decision-making capacity with illness progression. Adequate knowledge surrounding PC can influence the willingness of patients and families to accept PC (Cardenas et al., 2022; Myint et al., 2021) and thus information regarding PC should be communicated early in disease trajectory, such as at the time of diagnosis. Although there is not a reliable prognostication tool for dementia, The Gold Standards Framework states that early identification of patients in the final stage of life is important for high quality care and for end of life planning (The Gold Standards Framework, 2022). Since there are no curative or effective treatments for dementia, symptom management is a main goal which intensifies at the end of life (Sampson et al., 2011). Patients are faced with a myriad of symptoms, including pain, dyspnea, behaviour changes as a result of progressive cognitive impairment, and anxiety, which should not be underestimated. A commonly used scale for dementia illness trajectory is the GDS, or Reisberg scale, which can be seen in Table 1. Utilizing a scale for tracking the progression of illness may also be useful for healthcare providers to assess the needs of their patients.

PC will benefit all involved parties, including the patient, family, caregivers, and healthcare system. Its timely integration will lead to improvement of quality of the remaining life and better symptom control, leading to a good death, alleviation of caregiver distress, prevention of repeated emergency room visits, and reduction in burden on the healthcare system. Eliminating polypharmacy by deprescribing certain medications, including cognitive enhancers, neuroleptics, antihypertensives, vitamins, and supplements, is appropriate near the end of life to minimize pill burden and medication side effects. There is no benefit in artificial feeding for dementia patients at the end of life as the risk of aspiration events is almost the same with or without a feeding tube (I. Li, 2002), and there is a lack of nutritional advantage (Harris, 2007).

Financial benefits for the healthcare system are not to be underestimated. Deprescribing will reduce pharmacy costs. Dementia patients who receive PC have significantly reduced usage of medical services, medical department visits, and frequency of hospitalization (Chu et al., 2020).

Despite the multiple benefits of PC in dementia, unfortunately there are barriers associated with accessing these services due to age-related inequalities. Efforts to mitigate these barriers are essential to offer better quality of life and care for patients with dementia.

Future Research

Since the existing standard of care does not include consultation with PC when a patient is diagnosed with dementia (Murphy et al., 2016), there is need for further research to elicit the moving pieces that would be required to establish such a system and allow for timely referral to PC. The SQ is an approach that may be utilized to trigger timely PC consultation, which is known to have suitable specificity (ie. identification of true positives), despite its poor sensitivity (high rate of false positives) (Downar et al., 2017). Qualitative research exploring the perspectives of patients with dementia, their caregivers, and family members may be advantageous in understanding the needs of each party involved.

It may be useful to explore patient and caregiver thoughts on the perceived benefits of ACP in patients with dementia, to help with optimization of the process, improve comfort levels with ACP, and promote timely referral to PC. Lack of confidence in healthcare providers requires further exploration from the perspective of patients and caregivers. This can also help to identify existing gaps, enhance public education about PC, and lead to better acceptance of PC by patients and caregivers in advanced stages of the illness.

As it stands, there are few dependable tools for physicians to use for prognostication in dementia, and the current methods have marked limitations. Therefore, there is a need for the development of novel tools for more accurate prognostication in dementia, which would assist with the timely integration of PC and would lead to the creation of new models of care for this population. Additionally, more studies are needed on the incorporation of the frailty index in prognostication.

There is also no current model existing outlining the role of PC in dementia. Compared to cancer treatment, there is a lack of systemization in PC for dementia patients (Iliffe et al., 2013). More studies are needed to test and optimize the models used in the COMPASSION Intervention and IMPACT project, to standardize provision of PC in dementia.

Further research on the development of more robust guidelines for deprescribing practice in dementia would be beneficial for physicians and patients. Benefits of deprescribing in dementia patients and healthcare savings could be evaluated in multiple settings.

Although quality PC is of immense benefit for patients with dementia, there are multiple barriers in the healthcare system that hinder its provision. These include staffing shortages, limited staff time, and minimal funding. The system overall requires restructuring to prioritize PC in dementia, and further effort is required to ensure accessibility for older patients with dementia to PC services.

Lastly, further research is required to develop education programs outlining the role of PC for those suffering with dementia at the community level to ameliorate the stigma associated with PC. Current ongoing work by Carter et al. (2021) in the development of a digital game to educate the public about dementia has yielded positive results (Carter et al., 2021), and there is a great need for development of digestible and enjoyable educational resources, similar to this one. Investigation of the perspectives of patients, caregivers, and healthcare providers are invaluable in determining the types of resources that would be useful to develop, and how they can be optimized and disseminated to best reach the community.

Conclusion

Dementia is a complex, multifaceted terminal illness that significantly affects the lives of patients and their caregivers. Models for prognostication are limited. There is no existent cure and treatment is challenging. The multiple and varied needs of dementia patients are best-suited for management through a personalized and multidisciplinary approach.

ACP is crucial in dementia to educate patients on the illness trajectory and align treatment with their values and preferences. ACP needs to be introduced at the time of diagnosis or in earlier stages of illness trajectory as patients often lose cognitive abilities with disease progression. A personalized approach involving timely integrated PC can be curated to address physical, psychological, and cognitive domains of care in those affected by dementia. Deprescribing is of paramount importance to reduce pill burden and unfavourable side effects in this frail population, especially at the end of life. Overall, implementation of evidence-based models of care is needed to assist physicians and healthcare teams in providing care for dementia patients.

Despite dementia being a terminal illness, it is not always regarded as such, thus obscuring the timely integration of PC in this population. There is an imminent need for education about the benefits of PC in dementia for the public and healthcare providers. For caregivers, this knowledge may lead to willingness to accept PC, reduction of caregiver burden, and improvement of quality of life for all parties involved. Eliminating the stigma that aligns PC with death has been a longstanding challenge, which may be especially exaggerated in dementia as it is not always viewed as a terminal illness. Illness trajectory is poorly understood, and adequate training for healthcare professionals is crucial. Resource shortages in multiple countries prevent LTC facilities from providing the best quality of care to dementia patients. Although challenging, resource reallocation for the development of adequate training programs for administration of appropriate care is needed for providing a higher standard of PC for dementia patients.

Conclusively, implementing PC earlier in dementia disease trajectory provides multiple benefits to patients, caregivers, healthcare providers, and the healthcare system as a whole. Further efforts are required to overcome barriers and shift the current standard of care in dementia to include PC services.

References

Abel, J. (2013). Withdrawing life-extending drugs at the end of life: Stopping Drugs. *Prescriber, 24*(13–16), 17–20. https://doi.org/10.1002/psb.1083

Achterberg, W. P., Pieper, M. J., van Dalen-Kok, A. H., de Waal, M. W., Husebo, B. S., Lautenbacher, S., Kunz, M., Scherder, E. J., & Corbett, A. (2013). Pain management in patients with dementia. *Clinical Interventions in Aging, 8*, 1471–1482. https://doi.org/10.2147/CIA.S36739

Alzheimer Society of Canada. (2019, May). *Dementia and Responsive Behaviours*. https://alzheimer.ca/sites/default/files/documents/conversations_dementia-and-responsive-behaviours.pdf

Anantapong, K., Barrado-Martín, Y., Nair, P., Rait, G., Smith, C.H., Moore, K.J., Manthorpe, J., Sampson, E.L., & Davies, N. (2021). Abstract D-11: Perspectives of Older People Living with Mild Dementia about Eating and Drinking Problems at the Later Stages of Dementia: A Qualitative Study. In Abstracts from the 17th World Congress of the EAPC 2021. *Palliative Medicine, 35*(1_suppl), 41.

Anderson, F., Downing, G. M., Hill, J., Casorso, L., & Lerch, N. (1996). Palliative performance scale (PPS): A new tool. *Journal of Palliative Care, 12*(1), 5–11.

Araw, M., Kozikowski, A., Sison, C., Mir, T., Saad, M., Corrado, L., Pekmezaris, R., & Wolf-Klein, G. (2015). Does a palliative care consult decrease the cost of caring for hospitalized patients with dementia? *Palliative & Supportive Care, 13*(6), 1535–1540. https://doi.org/10.1017/S1478951513000795

Arcand, M. (2015). End-of-life issues in advanced dementia: Part 2: management of poor nutritional intake, dehydration, and pneumonia.

Canadian Family Physician Medecin De Famille Canadien, *61*(4), 337–341.

Ballard, C., Lana, M. M., Theodoulou, M., Douglas, S., McShane, R., Jacoby, R., Kossakowski, K., Yu, L.-M., & Juszczak, E. (2008). A randomised, blinded, placebo-controlled trial in dementia patients continuing or stopping neuroleptics (the DART-AD Trial). *PLoS Medicine*, *5*(4), 587–600.

Batzlaff, C. M., Karpman, C., Afessa, B., & Benzo, R. P. (2014). Predicting 1-Year Mortality Rate for Patients Admitted With an Acute Exacerbation of Chronic Obstructive Pulmonary Disease to an Intensive Care Unit: An Opportunity for Palliative Care. *Mayo Clinic Proceedings*, *89*(5), 638–643. https://doi.org/10.1016/j.mayocp.2013.12.004

Berrio, M. W., & Levesque, M. E. (1996). Advance directives. Most patients don't have one. Do yours? *The American Journal of Nursing*, *96*(8), 24–28; quiz 29.

Booker, R., & Bruce, A. (2020). Palliative sedation and medical assistance in dying: Distinctly different or simply semantics? *Nursing Inquiry*, *27*(1), e12321. https://doi.org/10.1111/nin.12321

Borges, M. K., Canevelli, M., Cesari, M., & Aprahamian, I. (2019). Frailty as a Predictor of Cognitive Disorders: A Systematic Review and Meta-Analysis. *Frontiers in Medicine*, *6*, 26. https://doi.org/10.3389/fmed.2019.00026

Bravo, G., Rodrigue, C., Arcand, M., Downie, J., Dubois, M.-F., Kaasalainen, S., Hertogh, C. M., Pautex, S., Van den Block, L., & Trottier, L. (2018). Quebec physicians' perspectives on medical aid in dying for incompetent patients with dementia. *Canadian Journal of Public Health = Revue Canadienne de Santé Publique*, *109*(5–6), 729–739. https://doi.org/10.17269/s41997-018-0115-9

Brown, M. A., Sampson, E. L., Jones, L., & Barron, A. M. (2013). Prognostic indicators of 6-month mortality in elderly people with advanced dementia: A systematic review. *Palliative Medicine*, *27*(5), 389–400. https://doi.org/10.1177/0269216312465649

Bullain, S. S., Corrada, M. M., Shah, B. A., Mozaffar, F. H., Panzenboeck, M., & Kawas, C. H. (2013). Poor Physical Performance and Dementia in the Oldest Old. *JAMA Neurology*, *70*(1), 107–113. https://doi.org/10.1001/jamaneurol.2013.583

Burge, F. I., Lawson, B. J., Johnston, G. M., & Grunfeld, E. (2008). A Population-based Study of Age Inequalities in Access to Palliative Care Among Cancer Patients. *Medical Care*, *46*(12), 1203–1211. https://doi.org/10.1097/MLR.0b013e31817d931d

Carter, G., Brown Wilson, C., Mitchell, G. Abstract A-04: Developing a Digital Game to Improve Public Perception of Dementia. (2021). In Abstracts from the 17th World Congress of the EAPC 2021. *Palliative Medicine*, *35*(1_suppl), 30-21. https://doi.org/10.1177/02692163211035909

Canadian Institute for Health Information. (n.d.). *Palliative and end-of-life care [report]*. Retrieved 26 February 2023, from https://www.cihi.ca/en/dementia-in-canada/spotlight-on-dementia-issues/palliative-and-end-of-life-care

Cardenas, V., Rahman, A., Zhu, Y., & Enguidanos, S. (2022). Reluctance to Accept Palliative Care and Recommendations for Improvement: Findings From Semi-Structured Interviews With Patients and Caregivers. *The American Journal of Hospice & Palliative Care*, *39*(2), 189–195. https://doi.org/10.1177/10499091211012605

Chu, C.-P., Huang, C.-Y., Kuo, C.-J., Chen, Y.-Y., Chen, C.-T., Yang, T.-W., & Liu, H.-C. (2020). Palliative care for nursing home patients with dementia: Service evaluation and risk factors of mortality. *BMC*

Palliative Care, 19(1), 122. https://doi.org/10.1186/s12904-020-00627-9

Continua Hospice Learning. (n.d.). *Hospice Care: How To Use The Karnofsky Performance Scale*. Retrieved 26 February 2023, from https://continuagroup.com/article/guidelines-for-use-the-karnofsky-performance-scale/

Cooper, C., Lodwick, R., Walters, K., Raine, R., Manthorpe, J., Iliffe, S., & Petersen, I. (2016). Observational cohort study: Deprivation and access to anti-dementia drugs in the UK. *Age and Ageing, 45*(1), 148–154. https://doi.org/10.1093/ageing/afv154

Crawley, S., West, E., Kupeli, N., & Moore, K. (2021). Abstract C-03: Predictors of Pre-death and Post Death Grief in Family Carers of People with Dementia. A Systematic Review. In Abstracts from the 17th World Congress of the EAPC 2021. *Palliative Medicine, 35*(1_suppl), 40. https://doi.org/10.1177/02692163211035909

Curtin, D., Jennings, E., Daunt, R., Curtin, S., Randles, M., Gallagher, P., & O'Mahony, D. (2020). Deprescribing in Older People Approaching End of Life: A Randomized Controlled Trial Using STOPPFrail Criteria. *Journal of the American Geriatrics Society, 68*(4), 762–769. https://doi.org/10.1111/jgs.16278

de Oliveira, A. M., Radanovic, M., de Mello, P. C. H., Buchain, P. C., Vizzotto, A. D. B., Celestino, D. L., Stella, F., Piersol, C. V., & Forlenza, O. V. (2015). Nonpharmacological Interventions to Reduce Behavioral and Psychological Symptoms of Dementia: A Systematic Review. *BioMed Research International, 2015*, 218980. https://doi.org/10.1155/2015/218980

Dolara, A. (2020). Deprescribing: A challenge for clinical cardiologists. *Acta Cardiologica, 75*(4), 295–297. https://doi.org/10.1080/00015385.2019.1593286

Downar, J., Goldman, R., Pinto, R., Englesakis, M., & Adhikari, N. K. J. (2017). The "surprise question" for predicting death in seriously ill patients: A systematic review and meta-analysis. *CMAJ : Canadian Medical Association Journal*, *189*(13), E484–E493. https://doi.org/10.1503/cmaj.160775

Easterling, C. S., & Robbins, E. (2008). Dementia and dysphagia. *Geriatric Nursing (New York, N.Y.)*, *29*(4), 275–285. https://doi.org/10.1016/j.gerinurse.2007.10.015

Ekbom, T., Lindholm, L. H., Odén, A., Dahlöf, B., Hansson, L., Wester, P. O., & Scherstén, B. (1994). A 5-year prospective, observational study of the withdrawal of antihypertensive treatment in elderly people. *Journal of Internal Medicine*, *235*(6), 581–588. https://doi.org/10.1111/j.1365-2796.1994.tb01265.x

Empeño, J., Raming, N. T. J., Irwin, S. A., Nelesen, R. A., & Lloyd, L. S. (2011). The hospice caregiver support project: Providing support to reduce caregiver stress. *Journal of Palliative Medicine*, *14*(5), 593–597. https://doi.org/10.1089/jpm.2010.0520

Forbes, D. A. (2018). Integrated Knowledge Translation Strategies that Enhance the Lives of Persons with Dementia and Their Family Caregivers. *Online Journal of Rural Nursing and Health Care*, *18*(1), 209–238. https://doi.org/10.14574/ojrnhc.v18i1.512

Freund-Levi, Y., Jedenius, E., Tysen-Bäckström, A. C., Lärksäter, M., Wahlund, L.-O., & Eriksdotter, M. (2014). Galantamine versus risperidone treatment of neuropsychiatric symptoms in patients with probable dementia: An open randomized trial. *The American Journal of Geriatric Psychiatry: Official Journal of the American Association for Geriatric Psychiatry*, *22*(4), 341–348. https://doi.org/10.1016/j.jagp.2013.05.005

Gardiner, C., Cobb, M., Gott, M., & Ingleton, C. (2011). Barriers to providing palliative care for older people in acute hospitals. *Age and Ageing*, *40*(2), 233–238. https://doi.org/10.1093/ageing/afq172

Garfinkel, D. (2018). Poly-de-prescribing to treat polypharmacy: Efficacy and safety. *Therapeutic Advances in Drug Safety*, *9*(1), 25–43. https://doi.org/10.1177/2042098617736192

Gillam, J., Davies, N., Aworinde, J., Yorganci, E., Anderson, J., & Evans, C. (2021). Abstract A-09: Implementation of eHealth Interventions to Support Assessment and Decision Making for Residents with Dementia in Care Homes: A Systematic Review. In Abstracts from the 17th World Congress of the EAPC 2021. *Palliative Medicine*, *35*(1_suppl), 31-32. https://doi.org/10.1177/02692163211035909

Goyal, P., Anderson, T. S., Bernacki, G. M., Marcum, Z. A., Orkaby, A. R., Kim, D., Zullo, A., Krishnaswami, A., Weissman, A., Steinman, M. A., & Rich, M. W. (2020). Physician Perspectives on Deprescribing Cardiovascular Medications for Older Adults. *Journal of the American Geriatrics Society*, *68*(1), 78–86. https://doi.org/10.1111/jgs.16157

Gruber-Baldini, A. L., Zimmerman, S., Boustani, M., Watson, L. C., Williams, C. S., & Reed, P. S. (2005). Characteristics associated with depression in long-term care residents with dementia. *The Gerontologist*, *45 Spec No 1*(1), 50–55. https://doi.org/10.1093/geront/45.suppl_1.50

Harris, D. (2007). Forget me not: Palliative care for people with dementia. *Postgraduate Medical Journal*, *83*(980), 362–366. https://doi.org/10.1136/pgmj.2006.052936

Harrison Dening, K. (2018). Advance care planning and people with dementia. In *Thomas K, Lobo B, Detering K (Eds.), Advance care planning in end of life care* (2nd ed., pp. 181–194). Oxford University Press.

Harrison Dening, K., Sampson, E. L., & De Vries, K. (2019). Advance care planning in dementia: Recommendations for healthcare professionals. *Palliative Care*, *12*, 1178224219826579. https://doi.org/10.1177/1178224219826579

Harrison, J. K., Van Der Wardt, V., Conroy, S. P., Stott, D. J., Dening, T., Gordon, A. L., Logan, P., Welsh, T. J., Taggar, J., Harwood, R., & Gladman, J. R. F. (2016). New horizons: The management of hypertension in people with dementia. *Age and Ageing*, *45*(6), 740–746. https://doi.org/10.1093/ageing/afw155

Hendriks, S. A., Smalbrugge, M., Galindo-Garre, F., Hertogh, C. M. P. M., & van der Steen, J. T. (2015). From Admission to Death: Prevalence and Course of Pain, Agitation, and Shortness of Breath, and Treatment of These Symptoms in Nursing Home Residents With Dementia. *Journal of the American Medical Directors Association*, *16*(6), 475–481. https://doi.org/10.1016/j.jamda.2014.12.016

Hendriks, S. A., Smalbrugge, M., Hertogh, C. M. P. M., & van der Steen, J. T. (2017). Changes in Care Goals and Treatment Orders Around the Occurrence of Health Problems and Hospital Transfers in Dementia: A Prospective Study. *Journal of the American Geriatrics Society*, *65*(4), 769–776. https://doi.org/10.1111/jgs.14667

Hill, E., Savundranayagam, M. Y., Zecevic, A., & Kloseck, M. (2018). Staff Perspectives of Barriers to Access and Delivery of Palliative Care for Persons With Dementia in Long-Term Care. *American Journal of Alzheimer's Disease and Other Dementias*, *33*(5), 284–291. https://doi.org/10.1177/1533317518765124

Hoe, J., Hancock, G., Livingston, G., Woods, B., Challis, D., & Orrell, M. (2009). CHANGES IN THE QUALITY OF LIFE OF PEOPLE WITH DEMENTIA LIVING IN CARE HOMES. *Alzheimer Disease and Associated Disorders*, *23*(3), 285–290. https://doi.org/10.1097/WAD.0b013e318194fc1e

Holmes, H. M., Sachs, G. A., Shega, J. W., Hougham, G. W., Cox Hayley, D., & Dale, W. (2008). Integrating palliative medicine into the care of persons with advanced dementia: Identifying appropriate medication use. *Journal of the American Geriatrics Society*, *56*(7), 1306–1311. https://doi.org/10.1111/j.1532-5415.2008.01741.x

Howes, L. G. (2014). Cardiovascular Effects of Drugs Used to Treat Alzheimer's Disease. *Drug Safety*, *37*(6), 391–395. https://doi.org/10.1007/s40264-014-0161-z

Hughes, J. C., Jolley, D., Jordan, A., & Sampson, E. L. (2007). Palliative care in dementia: Issues and evidence. *Advances in Psychiatric Treatment*, *13*(4), 251–260. https://doi.org/10.1192/apt.bp.106.003442

Hugo, J., & Ganguli, M. (2014). Dementia and cognitive impairment: Epidemiology, diagnosis, and treatment. *Clinics in Geriatric Medicine*, *30*(3), 421–442. https://doi.org/10.1016/j.cger.2014.04.001

Husebo, B. S., Ballard, C., Cohen-Mansfield, J., Seifert, R., & Aarsland, D. (2014). The response of agitated behavior to pain management in persons with dementia. *The American Journal of Geriatric Psychiatry: Official Journal of the American Association for Geriatric Psychiatry*, *22*(7), 708–717. https://doi.org/10.1016/j.jagp.2012.12.006

Iliffe, S., Davies, N., Vernooij-Dassen, M., van Riet Paap, J., Sommerbakk, R., Mariani, E., Jaspers, B., Radbruch, L., Manthorpe, J., Maio, L., Haugen, D., Engels, Y., & for the IMPACT research team. (2013). Modelling the landscape of palliative care for people with dementia: A European mixed methods study. *BMC Palliative Care*, *12*(1), 30. https://doi.org/10.1186/1472-684X-12-30

Jackson, S., Ham, R. J., & Wilkinson, D. (2004). The safety and tolerability of donepezil in patients with Alzheimer's disease. *British Journal of*

Clinical Pharmacology, *58*(Suppl 1), 1–8.

https://doi.org/10.1111/j.1365-2125.2004.01848.x

Jones, L., Candy, B., Davis, S., Elliott, M., Gola, A., Harrington, J., Kupeli, N., Lord, K., Moore, K., Scott, S., Vickerstaff, V., Omar, R. Z., King, M., Leavey, G., Nazareth, I., & Sampson, E. L. (2016). Development of a model for integrated care at the end of life in advanced dementia: A whole systems UK-wide approach. *Palliative Medicine*, *30*(3), 279–295.

https://doi.org/10.1177/0269216315605447

Kwak, Y. T., Yang, Y., & Koo, M.-S. (2017). Anxiety in Dementia. *Dementia and Neurocognitive Disorders*, *16*(2), 33–39. https://doi.org/10.12779/dnd.2017.16.2.33

Leung, J. G. (2014). Donepezil-induced mania. *The Consultant Pharmacist: The Journal of the American Society of Consultant Pharmacists*, *29*(3), 191–195.

https://doi.org/10.4140/TCP.n.2014.191

Li, I. (2002). Feeding Tubes in Patients with Severe Dementia. *American Family Physician*, *65*(8), 1605.

Li, M., Huang, Y., Liu, Z., Shen, R., Chen, H., Ma, C., Zhang, T., Li, S., & Prince, M. (2020). The association between frailty and incidence of dementia in Beijing: Findings from 10/66 dementia research group population-based cohort study. *BMC Geriatrics*, *20*(1), 138.

https://doi.org/10.1186/s12877-020-01539-2

Lindskog, M., Tavelin, B., & Lundström, S. (2015). Old age as risk indicator for poor end-of-life care quality—A population-based study of cancer deaths from the Swedish Register of Palliative Care. *European Journal of Cancer (Oxford, England: 1990)*, *51*(10), 1331–1339. https://doi.org/10.1016/j.ejca.2015.04.001

Linklater, G., Barton, S., Lawton, S., & Pang, D. (2011). The use of the Palliative Performance in individuals with dementia and frailty. *Age*

and Ageing, *40*(eLetters Supplement).
https://doi.org/10.1093/ageing/el_154

Linklater, G., Lawton, S., Fielding, S., Macaulay, L., Carroll, D., & Pang, D. (2012). Introducing the Palliative Performance Scale to clinicians: The Grampian experience. *BMJ Supportive & Palliative Care*, *2*(2), 121–126. https://doi.org/10.1136/bmjspcare-2011-000133

Luengo-Fernandez, R., Leal, J., & Gray, A. M. (2011). Cost of dementia in the pre-enlargement countries of the European Union. *Journal of Alzheimer's Disease: JAD*, *27*(1), 187–196. https://doi.org/10.3233/JAD-2011-102019

Mantelli, S., Jungo, K. T., Rozsnyai, Z., Reeve, E., Luymes, C. H., Poortvliet, R. K. E., Chiolero, A., Rodondi, N., Gussekloo, J., & Streit, S. (2018). How general practitioners would deprescribe in frail oldest-old with polypharmacy—The LESS study. *BMC Family Practice*, *19*(1), 169. https://doi.org/10.1186/s12875-018-0856-9

Martinsson, L., Lundström, S., & Sundelöf, J. (2018). Quality of end-of-life care in patients with dementia compared to patients with cancer: A population-based register study. *PloS One*, *13*(7), e0201051. https://doi.org/10.1371/journal.pone.0201051

McGovern, J. (2015). Living Better With Dementia: Strengths-Based Social Work Practice and Dementia Care. *Social Work in Health Care*, *54*(5), 408–421.
https://doi.org/10.1080/00981389.2015.1029661

Mimica, N., & Presecki, P. (2009). Side effects of approved antidementives. *Psychiatria Danubina*, *21*(1), 108–113.

Minaglia, C., Giannotti, C., Boccardi, V., Mecocci, P., Serafini, G., Odetti, P., & Monacelli, F. (2019). Cachexia and advanced dementia. *Journal of Cachexia, Sarcopenia and Muscle*, *10*(2), 263–277. https://doi.org/10.1002/jcsm.12380

Mitchell, G. K., Senior, H. E., Rhee, J. J., Ware, R. S., Young, S., Teo, P. C., Murray, S., Boyd, K., & Clayton, J. M. (2018). Using intuition or a formal palliative care needs assessment screening process in general practice to predict death within 12 months: A randomised controlled trial. *Palliative Medicine*, *32*(2), 384–394. https://doi.org/10.1177/0269216317698621

Mitchell, S. L., Miller, S. C., Teno, J. M., Davis, R. B., & Shaffer, M. L. (2010). The Advanced Dementia Prognostic Tool (ADEPT): A Risk Score to Estimate Survival in Nursing Home Residents with Advanced Dementia. *Journal of Pain and Symptom Management*, *40*(5), 639–651. https://doi.org/10.1016/j.jpainsymman.2010.02.014

Moore, K. J., Candy, B., Davis, S., Gola, A., Harrington, J., Kupeli, N., Vickerstaff, V., King, M., Leavey, G., Nazareth, I., Omar, R. Z., Jones, L., & Sampson, E. L. (2017). Implementing the compassion intervention, a model for integrated care for people with advanced dementia towards the end of life in nursing homes: A naturalistic feasibility study. *BMJ Open*, *7*(6), e015515. https://doi.org/10.1136/bmjopen-2016-015515

Murphy, E., Froggatt, K., Connolly, S., O'Shea, E., Sampson, E. L., Casey, D., & Devane, D. (2016). Palliative care interventions in advanced dementia. *The Cochrane Database of Systematic Reviews*, *2016*(12), CD011513. https://doi.org/10.1002/14651858.CD011513.pub2

Murray, S. A., Kendall, M., Boyd, K., & Sheikh, A. (2005). Illness trajectories and palliative care. *BMJ : British Medical Journal*, *330*(7498), 1007–1011.

Murray, S. A., & Sheikh, A. (2008). Care for all at the end of life. *BMJ : British Medical Journal*, *336*(7650), 958–959. https://doi.org/10.1136/bmj.39535.491238.94

Myint, A. T., Tiraphat, S., Jayasvasti, I., Hong, S. A., & Kasemsup, V. (2021). Factors Influencing the Willingness of Palliative Care

Utilization among the Older Population with Active Cancers: A Case Study in Mandalay, Myanmar. *International Journal of Environmental Research and Public Health*, *18*(15), 7887. https://doi.org/10.3390/ijerph18157887

Nakanishi, A., Cuthbertson, L., & Chase, J. (2021). Advance Requests for Medical Assistance in Dying in Dementia: A Survey Study of Dementia Care Specialists. *Canadian Geriatrics Journal*, *24*(2), 82–95. https://doi.org/10.5770/cgj.24.496

National Institute for Health and Care Excellence. (2018). *Dementia: Assessment, management and support for people living with dementia and their carers*. National Institute for Health and Care Excellence (NICE). http://www.ncbi.nlm.nih.gov/books/NBK513207/

NIH National Institute on Aging. (2017, May 16). *What Happens to the Brain in Alzheimer's Disease?* National Institute on Aging. https://www.nia.nih.gov/health/what-happens-brain-alzheimers-disease

NIH National Institute on Aging. (2022, October 31). *Advance Care Planning: Advance Directives for Health Care*. National Institute on Aging. https://www.nia.nih.gov/health/advance-care-planning-advance-directives-health-care

Palagyi, A., Keay, L., Harper, J., Potter, J., & Lindley, R. I. (2016). Barricades and brickwalls – a qualitative study exploring perceptions of medication use and deprescribing in long-term care. *BMC Geriatrics*, *16*(1), 15. https://doi.org/10.1186/s12877-016-0181-x

Pandpazir, M., & Tajari, M. (2019). The application of palliative care in dementia. *Journal of Family Medicine and Primary Care*, *8*(2), 347–351. https://doi.org/10.4103/jfmpc.jfmpc_105_18

Parker, D. (2021). Abstract PL3: Meeting the Challenge of Dementia Care in the Future. In: Abstracts from the 17th World Congress of the

EAPC 2021. *Palliative Medicine*, *35*(1_suppl), 24. https://doi.org/10.1177/02692163211035909

Parsons, C., Hughes, C. M., Passmore, A. P., & Lapane, K. L. (2010). Withholding, Discontinuing and Withdrawing Medications in Dementia Patients at the End of Life. *Drugs & Aging*, *27*(6), 435–449. https://doi.org/10.2165/11536760-000000000-00000

Parsons, C., McCorry, N., Murphy, K., Byrne, S., O'Sullivan, D., O'Mahony, D., Passmore, P., Patterson, S., & Hughes, C. (2014). Assessment of factors that influence physician decision making regarding medication use in patients with dementia at the end of life. *International Journal of Geriatric Psychiatry*, *29*(3), 281–290. https://doi.org/10.1002/gps.4006

Payne, M., & Morley, J. E. (2018). Dysphagia, Dementia and Frailty. *The Journal of Nutrition, Health & Aging*, *22*(5), 562–565. https://doi.org/10.1007/s12603-018-1033-5

Phillipson, L., Goodenough, B., Reis, S., & Fleming, R. (2016). Applying Knowledge Translation Concepts and Strategies in Dementia Care Education for Health Professionals: Recommendations From a Narrative Literature Review. *The Journal of Continuing Education in the Health Professions*, *36*(1), 74–81. https://doi.org/10.1097/CEH.0000000000000028

Pope, T. M. (2021). Medical Aid in Dying and Dementia Directives. *Canadian Journal of Bioethics*, *4*(2), 82–86.

Pype, P., Mertens, F., Helewaut, F., D'Hulster, B., & Sutter, A. D. (2018). Potentially inappropriate medication in primary care at the end of life: A mixed-method study. *Acta Clinica Belgica*, *73*(3), 213–219. https://doi.org/10.1080/17843286.2017.1410606

Reeve, E., Farrell, B., Thompson, W., Herrmann, N., Sketris, I., Magin, P. J., Chenoweth, L., Gorman, M., Quirke, L., Bethune, G., & Hilmer, S. N. (2019). Deprescribing cholinesterase inhibitors and memantine in dementia: Guideline summary. *Medical Journal of Australia*, *210*(4), 174–179. https://doi.org/10.5694/mja2.50015

Reeve, E., Shakib, S., Hendrix, I., Roberts, M. S., & Wiese, M. D. (2014). The benefits and harms of deprescribing. *Medical Journal of Australia*, *201*(7), 386–389. https://doi.org/10.5694/mja13.00200

Reisberg, B., Ferris, S. H., de Leon, M. J., & Crook, T. (1982). The Global Deterioration Scale for assessment of primary degenerative dementia. *The American Journal of Psychiatry*, *139*(9), 1136–1139. https://doi.org/10.1176/ajp.139.9.1136

Rosenwax, L., Spilsbury, K., Arendts, G., McNamara, B., & Semmens, J. (2015). Community-based palliative care is associated with reduced emergency department use by people with dementia in their last year of life: A retrospective cohort study. *Palliative Medicine*, *29*(8), 727–736. https://doi.org/10.1177/0269216315576309

Sampson, E. L., Anderson, J. E., Candy, B., Davies, N., Ellis-Smith, C., Gola, A., Harding, R., Kenten, C., Kupeli, N., Mead, S., Moore, K. J., Omar, R. Z., Sleeman, K. E., Stewart, R., Ward, J., Warren, J. D., & Evans, C. J. (2020). Empowering Better End-of-Life Dementia Care (EMBED-Care): A mixed methods protocol to achieve integrated person-centred care across settings. *International Journal of Geriatric Psychiatry*, *35*(8), 820–832. https://doi.org/10.1002/gps.5251

Sampson, E. L., Jones, L., Thuné-Boyle, I. C., Kukkastenvehmas, R., King, M., Leurent, B., Tookman, A., & Blanchard, M. R. (2011). Palliative assessment and advance care planning in severe dementia: An exploratory randomized controlled trial of a complex intervention. *Palliative Medicine*, *25*(3), 197–209. https://doi.org/10.1177/0269216310391691

Sarbacker, G. B. (2014). Pain management in dementia. *US Pharm*, *39*(3), 39–43.

Schunk, M., Thomsen, J.-M, Streitwieser, S., Port, G., & Bausewein, C. (2021). Abstract PS03: Assessing palliative care needs in people with dementia using proxy measurement: validation of the Integrated Palliative care Outcome Scale for Dementia (IPOS-Dem) in German nursing homes. In Abstracts from the 17th World Congress of the EAPC 2021. *Palliative Medicine*, *35*(1_suppl), 8–9. https://doi.org/10.1177/02692163211035909

Schur, S., Weixler, D., Gabl, C., Kreye, G., Likar, R., Masel, E. K., Mayrhofer, M., Reiner, F., Schmidmayr, B., Kirchheiner, K., Watzke, H. H., & on behalf of the AUPACS (Austrian Palliative Care Study) Group. (2016). Sedation at the end of life—A nation-wide study in palliative care units in Austria. *BMC Palliative Care*, *15*(1), 50. https://doi.org/10.1186/s12904-016-0121-8

Senderovich, H., Ip, M. L., Berall, A., Karuza, J., Gordon, M., Binns, M., Wignarajah, S., Grossman, D., & Dunal, L. (2016). Therapeutic Touch® in a geriatric Palliative Care Unit – A retrospective review. *Complementary Therapies in Clinical Practice*, *24*, 134–138. https://doi.org/10.1016/j.ctcp.2016.06.002

Senderovich, H., & Retnasothie, S. (2020). A systematic review of the integration of palliative care in dementia management. *Palliative & Supportive Care*, *18*(4), 495–506. https://doi.org/10.1017/S1478951519000968

Sharp, E. S., & Gatz, M. (2011). The Relationship between Education and Dementia An Updated Systematic Review. *Alzheimer Disease and Associated Disorders*, *25*(4), 289–304. https://doi.org/10.1097/WAD.0b013e318211c83c

Steinhauser, K. E., Clipp, E. C., McNeilly, M., Christakis, N. A., McIntyre, L. M., & Tulsky, J. A. (2000). In search of a good death: Observations of patients, families, and providers. *Annals of Internal*

Medicine, 132(10), 825–832. https://doi.org/10.7326/0003-4819-132-10-200005160-00011

Sternberg, S., Bentur, N., & Shuldiner, J. (2014). Quality of care of older people living with advanced dementia in the community in Israel. *Journal of the American Geriatrics Society, 62*(2), 269–275. https://doi.org/10.1111/jgs.12655

The Gold Standards Framework (2022). Proactive Identification Guidance (PIG) The National GSF Centre's guidance for clinicians to support earlier identification of patients nearing the end of life, leading to improved proactive person-centred care. Available from: https://goldstandardsframework.org.uk/cdcontent/uploads/files/PIG/Proactive%20Identification%20Guidance%20v7%20(2022).pdf

Todd, A., Holmes, H., Pearson, S., Hughes, C., Andrew, I., Baker, L., & Husband, A. (2016). 'I don't think I'd be frightened if the statins went': A phenomenological qualitative study exploring medicines use in palliative care patients, carers and healthcare professionals. *BMC Palliative Care, 15*, 13. https://doi.org/10.1186/s12904-016-0086-7

van der Steen, J.T. (2021). Abstract PS11: Developing an evidence base to support advance care planning in dementia. In Abstracts from the 17th World Congress of the EAPC 2021. *Palliative Medicine, 35*(1_suppl), 14. https://doi.org/10.1177/02692163211035909

van der Steen, J. T., Lemos Dekker, N., Gijsberts, M.-J. H. E., Vermeulen, L. H., Mahler, M. M., & The, B. A.-M. (2017). Palliative care for people with dementia in the terminal phase: A mixed-methods qualitative study to inform service development. *BMC Palliative Care, 16*(1), 28. https://doi.org/10.1186/s12904-017-0201-4

Visiting Nurse Service of New York. (n.d.). *Palliative Performance Scale (PPS)*. Retrieved 28 February 2022, from https://www.vnsny.org/for-healthcare-professionals/referring-patients/hospice-palliative-care/palliative-performance-scale-pps/

Wang, C., Ji, X., Wu, X., Tang, Z., Zhang, X., Guan, S., Liu, H., & Fang, X. (2017). Frailty in Relation to the Risk of Alzheimer's Disease, Dementia, and Death in Older Chinese Adults: A Seven-Year Prospective Study. *The Journal of Nutrition, Health & Aging, 21*(6), 648–654. https://doi.org/10.1007/s12603-016-0798-7

Wang, Y., Xiao, L. D., Ullah, S., He, G.-P., & De Bellis, A. (2017). Evaluation of a nurse-led dementia education and knowledge translation programme in primary care: A cluster randomized controlled trial. *Nurse Education Today, 49*, 1–7. https://doi.org/10.1016/j.nedt.2016.10.016

Warden, V., Hurley, A. C., & Volicer, L. (2003). Development and psychometric evaluation of the Pain Assessment in Advanced Dementia (PAINAD) scale. *Journal of the American Medical Directors Association, 4*(1), 9–15. https://doi.org/10.1097/01.JAM.0000043422.31640.F7

Whitman, A., DeGregory, K., Morris, A., Mohile, S., & Ramsdale, E. (2018). Pharmacist-Led Medication Assessment and Deprescribing Intervention for Older Adults with Cancer and Polypharmacy: A Pilot Study. *Supportive Care in Cancer : Official Journal of the Multinational Association of Supportive Care in Cancer, 26*(12), 4105–4113. https://doi.org/10.1007/s00520-018-4281-3

Won, C. W. (2020). Diagnosis and Management of Frailty in Primary Health Care. *Korean Journal of Family Medicine, 41*(4), 207–213. https://doi.org/10.4082/kjfm.20.0122

Woods, D. L., Craven, R. F., & Whitney, J. (2005). The effect of therapeutic touch on behavioral symptoms of persons with dementia. *Alternative Therapies in Health and Medicine, 11*(1), 66–74.

World Health Organization. (2020, August 5). *Palliative care*.
https://www.who.int/news-room/fact-sheets/detail/palliative-care

World Health Organization. (2022, September 20). *Dementia*.
https://www.who.int/news-room/fact-sheets/detail/dementia

Yokomichi, N., Yamaguchi, T., Maeda, I., Mori, M., Imai, K., Shirado Naito, A., Yamaguchi, T., Terabayashi, T., Hiratsuka, Y., Hisanaga, T., & Morita, T. (2022). Effect of continuous deep sedation on survival in the last days of life of cancer patients: A multicenter prospective cohort study. *Palliative Medicine, 36*(1), 189–199. https://doi.org/10.1177/02692163211057754

Yorganci, E., Stewart, R., Sampson, E., & Sleeman, K. (2021). Abstract J-09: Patterns of Unplanned Hospital Admissions among People with Dementia: From Diagnosis to the End of Life. In Abstracts from the 17th World Congress of the EAPC 2021. *Palliative Medicine, 35*(1_suppl), 44. https://doi.org/10.1177/02692163211035909

More Books!

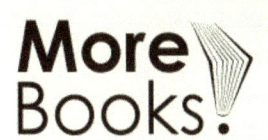

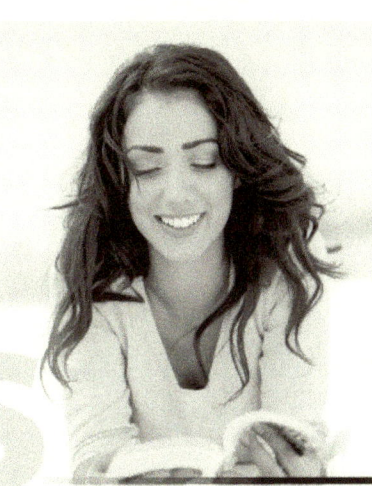

I want morebooks!

Buy your books fast and straightforward online - at one of world's fastest growing online book stores! Environmentally sound due to Print-on-Demand technologies.

Buy your books online at
www.morebooks.shop

Kaufen Sie Ihre Bücher schnell und unkompliziert online – auf einer der am schnellsten wachsenden Buchhandelsplattformen weltweit! Dank Print-On-Demand umwelt- und ressourcenschonend produziert.

Bücher schneller online kaufen
www.morebooks.shop

info@omniscriptum.com
www.omniscriptum.com

OMNIScriptum

www.ingramcontent.com/pod-product-compliance
Ingram Content Group UK Ltd.
Pitfield, Milton Keynes, MK11 3LW, UK
UKHW031304170225
4629UKWH00034B/336